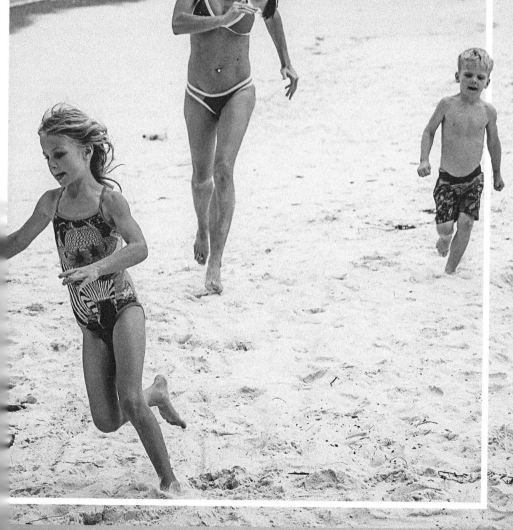

FIT, HEALTHY, HAPPY KIDS

A FOOD AND EXERCISE BLUEPRINT FOR CHILDREN UNDER 12

SHARNY ∞ JULIUS

www.sharnyandjulius.com

Fit, Healthy, Happy Kids by SHARNY &JULIUS
A food and exercise blueprint for children under 12

www.sharnyandjulius.com
email:sharnyandjulius@sharnyandjulius.com

Edited by: Laura Johnson

Cover Photography: sharnyandjulius

Typesetting and Design: sharnyandjulius

ISBN: 978-0-9923613-7-2

Contents

It was easy for us

Its very easy to look at kids these days and shake our heads. "you spend too much time on that bloody phone!" or "I used to play outside all day!" are easy to say, and they make sense.

Until we compare our childhood with that of our kids.

When we were kids, we used to play outside all day with the rest of the neighbourhood kids. Coming inside was scary, because mum would make us do the dishes!

Nowadays, kids aren't safe outside. The streets seem empty, predators stalk playgrounds, parks and bus stops. Every week there's a story about an abduction.

When we were kids, we'd have one TV in the entire house and dad would watch the news on it, or sport. Nowdays, everybody has a smart phone or computer or game console to keep them entertained. Most houses have more screens than bikes.

When we were kids, dad worked and mum only worked part time. Nowdays, mum and dad both have to work overtime just to keep up with expenses. They have less time to cook meals and rely on takeaway.

When we were kids, takeaway was a treat. Nowdays, home cooked meals are a treat.

When we were kids, food was food. Now, food is science. The science of addiction.

When we were kids, bread was baked by the local baker, meat was sourced by the local butcher and fruit was bought from the local farmers; who all lived in the same community. Now, all food gets shipped in bulk, from somewhere else, where manufacturers care about profit, not the community.

When we were kids, PE and sport were compulsory. Nowdays both are voluntary. Given the choice as kids, we too would have opted for sitting around doing nothing.

When we were kids, state sports teams were made up of local citizens. Community spirit is now just a relic of a bygone era.

The world our kids are growing up in is very different to the world we grew up in. The gap is so much wider than between us and our parents.

We grew up with nothing, so our parents worked hard to give us everything..

Our own generation's motto of "we deserve everything" has turned its greedy eyes to our kids, and they stand no chance. Right now, they are fending for themselves, in a world that sees only one outcome for them.

Victims of greed.

Unless us parents do something about it. We now need to work hard to protect our kids from our ourselves…

Thank you for buying this book

Thankyou, from both of us, and our kids, thankyou. If you are a *SharnyandJulius* collector, we've made sure that this book won't disappoint you. Finding time to read is hard these days, and we find most books on fitness to be like modern food; too stuffed full of junk to be of any value.

This book gets to the point fast, and will hopefully captivate you there for the few short hours it might take to read and then give you a good ol' slap on the back and a jump in your stride. By the time you are finished reading this book, you will have a blueprint for creating a perfectly balanced, healthy young child, and you will be excited about implementing it with them.

If this is your first *SharnyandJulius* book, we hope you like it and welcome to the family. Stick around for a bit, find us on our social media and our website, you'll find we're more than just a mum and dad; we're the voice of a community. A community that knows no geographic boundaries or racial segregation. We are a community whose defining factor is that we all care deeply and passionately about the health of our families.

Let's get into it.

Who this book is for

If you've got children between the ages of 1 and 12, this book has been written for you. We are currently writing the companion book, called *Fit, Healthy, Happy Teens*, which will help all parents of the most difficult species - the teenager - to get them as healthy as possible. Teenagers are completely different to young children, so if you have a teenage kid, by all means read this book - but know that we are working on a translation for the hormone generation.

If you do have kids between the ages of 1 and 12, you'll fall into one of two categories.

Your child is overweight and you're worried

If your child is already overweight, we're going to outline a plan for you to turn your little cherub into a health and exercise fanatic. Don't be alarmed, most kids these days are overweight, the problem is that most parents don't do anything about it. You have! By buying and reading this book, you are in the small percentage of parents who take themselves and their kids seriously enough to be worthy of the title "parent".

So sit back, relax; we've got your back.

You are worried that your child might become overweight

The world we live in is geared towards over consumption, everything and everybody wants your money, and to get it, they will seduce your innocent children. Fast food places give toys away with "food" so they can lure themselves a repeat customer.

Sounds a little harsh, but we're sure you know what we mean. Marketing companies know that the people with the most influence in our lives are our children, couple that with a child's exploratory innocence, and you can see why they put animals on candy packets.

We think it's sad and disgusting that they would be allowed to abuse the innocence of children like that, but it's the reality of the world we live in. If you don't actively teach your child about their environment, they will end up a victim of a marketing plan.

Prevention is much easier than cure, so I applaud you for wanting to get a good grip on your child's health well before anything adverse may happen. But be assured that what we are going to cover is not going to be hard. There's no weird stuff in here, just a realistic game plan for making your precious child into a shining beacon of health.

Our goal as parents

In July 2014, we will have our 5th child and will hopefully have more. We love kids, and we know how great a responsibility it is to have another human being in our absolute care. It's a scary thing too, if you choose to see it that way.

A lot of people try to be the same as they were before kids. They fight vehemently to keep their social lives intact, often getting the kids babysat so they can go out and party. But when it comes to our kids, there is no us and them. The selfishness of youth is over; we have children to care for, to nurture and to keep safe.

Maybe we're wrong, but we don't think about ourselves as individuals any more - for the next 18 years at least, we are a team. The Kieser team - we are our kids, our kids are us. With that said, we don't want to completely lose sight of the other important facet of our family, the love between husband and wife - so we created a purpose for ourselves as parents.

Our purpose as parents is to keep our children safe, and equip them with all the tools possible to become independent adults, unhindered by anything and that they choose us as their friends.

We'd like to take a moment to explain this in a bit more detail.

Firstly, **our purpose is to keep our kids safe**. Not only from obvious dangers like cars, dangerous dogs and sticking a knife in the toaster, but also from being influenced by others - a far more subtle threat. Allowing others to influence us, or being easily influenced is an enormous danger.

If you don't have a solid image of yourself, the marketing world will give you one - and it's version never sees you as a winner. We want our kids to have a solid perception of self.

We want them to become independent adults. A lot of parents we know put so much effort into shaping their children to become just like them, or better versions of themselves. A great example of this is the vicarious parents, we call them "show-mums" who have dreams of their kids attaining the highest levels of achievement possible in whatever they (the mums) could never achieve. Show-mums appoint themselves coach, life coach, mentor, judge, jury and owner of their child.

Children of show-mums grow up with no sense of who they really are. Lost, they cling to their parents for recognition and reward, or rebel completely to find out who they really are.

We don't want our kids to reach adulthood and not know who they are. We want to discover who they are by what they are attracted to and find unbridled joy in, not what we want them to do. It really doesn't matter what they make of their lives, as long as they are happy.

Happiness can only lead to positive things. We want our children to become independent of us. That means we don't want them to depend on us. Financially, emotionally or intellectually. We're just a couple of kids too!

One of the joys of being a parent is that your young children are so dependent on you. Imagining that one day they won't can be quite daunting. Some people hold things over their kids to make sure that when they leave the nest, they come back - like inheritance, like guilt.

We never want our kids to feel like they have to visit us or be around us; we want them to choose to. Not because we are their parents, but because if we weren't bound by the invisible strings of family, they would **still choose us as friends**.

This is a very powerful part of our purpose, because it makes us collaborators in their early lives, rather than dictators.

Our eldest son has just left home to start his studies, and while nothing can prepare you for the emptiness that is left behind, we can report that he is independent of us, and he has come home of his own volition very often. Not for money, not for food, but because we are his friends.

Absolve yourself of blame, but take responsibility

In the past 3 years, there has been a witch-hunt for who is at fault for this obesity epidemic. Fast food companies, government, schools, parents, everybody is blaming everybody else; but nobody wants to take responsibility.

Here's our take on it:

We. Don't. Care.

If you're standing on the edge of a flooding river, and a whole bunch of children fall in, whose fault is it? Is it your fault for not telling them to get back? Is it the school's fault for not educating them better on the dangers of flooded rivers? Is it the government's fault for not sealing off the slippery embankment?

We. Don't. Care.

We just want to save the kids. We're wasting time arguing about who is to blame when every second arguing could be spent saving a child from doom.

Childhood obesity is a flooded river, and our kids are all slipping in. The only thing that matters is getting them out.

If you've been beating yourself up with blame, stop it. We've got work to do. Only once your child is safe and healthy, can you go back and look at where you think you messed up. But in the meantime, we've got work to do.

Absolve yourself of blame. If you feel guilty, let it go. What's happened has happened. What you need to replace that blame or guilt with is responsibility.

Until someone puts their hand in the air and says, "I'll do it" nothing gets done. If we wait for someone else to solve the obesity epidemic, who knows how long that might be?

So let's put our hands in the air right now and say, "I'll do it."

And you know what the best part is? You only have to worry about your own family. If you worry about your family and we worry about our family; that makes two families that don't need any outside help.

If we can make our families into shining beacons of health and happiness, others will follow. It's not like we have to knock on doors to tell people how good our way of life is; they'll see it. They'll see it in our kids and in us. People will want what we've got, and they deserve it.

There is a massive shift happening right now. It's just a deep rumbling, but with a little push, it will soon be deafening.

People want to be healthy. The obsessive over consumptive selfish lifestyle has limitations, limitations that are being exposed daily. People are starting to realise that the freedom they think they have bought an illusion. The control they have over their lives is just borrowed.

Let's dig deeper.

Don't believe anything until you have proven it to yourself

Before you believe someone's weight loss cure or miracle, or food fad or anything for that matter, we find it best to find out the source and what the source gains from their theory.

Here are a few for you.

Myth: Engagement rings are an eternal sign on love

Truth: At the turn of the century, the DeBeers diamond mining company put up advertising posters around cities saying "if it's true love, seal it with a diamond." Engagement rings haven't been around for that long, and were created for profit alone; not for love.

Myth: To gain muscle you need to drink protein shakes.

Truth: Protein shakes are a substitute for lack of protein in a diet. A lot of bodybuilders and athletes don't take protein, and they exercise way more than we do, and still get great gains because the truth is that we get enough protein in a balanced diet anyway. Protein companies don't want you to know this, so they use steroid powered supermen to sell their protein powder.

Myth: Obesity is a disease

Truth: Obesity is a result of overeating, the disease is food addiction. Pharmaceutical companies can only get funding for drugs that treat a disease. Listing obesity as a disease will allow them to prescribe drugs for obesity. This doesn't cure the disease, it just treats the symptoms. Pharmaceutical drugs to reduce body fat do not cure overeating. People who are led to believe this end up broke, because they still buy and eat too much food, but now also buy their weight loss drugs.

Myth: The Heart Foundation is looking out for you

Truth: To get the heart foundation tick of approval, food companies have to pay. In business this is called licensing. The heart foundation is a brand, not a caring organisation. Next time you are in the supermarket, look for something with the heart foundation tick on it, then look at the ingredients list. Most of the ingredients are not even foods, they are chemicals.

If you look closely, most things you like to believe are just marketing. If you live in this modern world, and you think you have control, look again. When it comes to marketing, the truth is hidden.

Is sugar bad for you? Are you allergic to wheat? Is Garcinia Cambogia a miracle cure?

Find out for yourself. In the middle of this book, we'll go through a list of potential poisons that are currently quite trendy to avoid. We'll give you the research and ways to find out for yourself if you should in fact avoid them

Remember always, what works for us, may not work for you. Find out what works for you and then for each of your kids. In the mean time, don't believe anything until you have proven it yourself to be true.

While you ponder the rose coloured glasses marketers have given you, we'll delve into the first step to creating a family with healthy, happy kids - the healthy routine.

But before we look at your routine, we need to make sure that you've got your own head in the right place.

Get your own head right

A friend of ours who works long hours as an engineer in Sydney. His office is in the city centre, travel taking nearly 2 hours out of each workday. He lives outside the city, because he wants a back yard for his daughter.

Our friend leaves home before his daughter wakes up and comes home after she has gone back to sleep. The only time she ever sees him is on the weekend when he spends a lot of the time catching up on work.

We asked him one day if he regrets anything in his life and he said that he regrets not being able to see his daughter every day. We suggested he move closer to the city. "We wouldn't have a back yard any more."

"How often do you go in the back yard?"

"I mow it once a week."

"So you sacrifice 2 hours a day with your daughter for a back yard that nobody really uses."

Silence... then,

"We couldn't move anyway, it's too scummy in the city."

"So you sacrifice time with your daughter to live in a nice neighbourhood?" Then, pushing the bounds of friendship, "Why are you driving an Audi, why don't you drive a Hyundai?"

3 months later, he called to say he had moved to a country town on the West Coast for far less income than he was taking in the city, but here he drove 10 minutes to work, had a much bigger house and to top it off, he got rid of his Audi and bought a reliable Hyundai for a quarter of the price.

"When you're living in the city, you feel this pressure to be better, to not be a loser, so you work harder and you live in a more expensive neighbourhood and you drive a European car. But I thought to myself, what for? Who am I trying to impress? My daughter is growing up without a father, and she'll remember that. She won't remember what car I drove or whether she lived in the Northern Beaches, she'll only remember the time we spent together."

This is a great example of for change to happen, it has to start with you. Most young kids are a reflection of their environment, and you form a massive part of that environment.

If you work hard, are wealthy but unhealthy, trade in the fancy car for a more economical one, cut back on 2 or 3 hours a week and get your own self healthy.

If getting yourself healthy is the only thing you do, then this book has been worth every sleepless night it has taken us to write. Because your children love you so much that they will try so hard to become like you.

If you're a chain-smoking cola addict, you cannot expect them to be any different.

If you're a wellness fanatic who loves sport, your kids will mirror you.

Get your own head right, then we'll work on the kids.

If you feel like your head is not in the right place yet, read on, because a lot of these ideas are family wide changes - you'll see, it's not that difficult.

You've got this.

Part 1:
Food

Free yourself up with a routine

The most successful people on earth have one underlying attribute that they all share. A strict adherence to routine. We would go as far as to say that the more tight your daily routine, the more successful you are.

Think about the president of the USA. His routine is set in stone months in advance. He can't just kick back and let the woo-woo waves flow. That's for stoners and losers. Everything about his day is planned out months in advance. And it has to be.

Olympic athletes are the same; their training plan is mapped out for four years. Every meal is meticulously planned and designed to fit in with the end goal, years in advance. They too cannot afford to kick back and eat "whatever."

The poorest people you know have no routine. They just float through life on the poverty line, doing whatever they feel like moment to moment.

Obese people have the same attitude toward food. They'll leave home for work without packing lunch, or they'll wait until they are hungry to make a decision about what they are going to cook for dinner. Which ends up being "what am I going to eat for dinner?"

When they make that distinction – "what am I going to eat?" Instead of "what am I going to cook?" they open the door to fast food.

As we've said before, if you don't have a plan for your time/money/food...
you'll be at the mercy of someone else's plan for it.

A step by step guide to your own family routine

Cook as many meals at home as you can. Trusting someone else to feed you and your family leads to danger, so a healthy routine relies heavily on home cooked food. If you're not prepared to cook at home, then you'll need to hire a chef.

Step 1: Decide how many meals you are going to eat each week.

If you are going to eat 3 meals a day, that's 3 meals x 7 days. = 21 meals a week. If you choose to eat 6 meals a day, you'll need a plan for 42 meals every week.

We just eat 3 meals a day now. We used to eat 6, which is a good idea because you stop yourself from overeating at each meal. Now that our routine is fixed though, it's just easier to make 3 meals per day. 42 meals a week for a family of 7 just overwhelms us.

Step 2: Decide/calculate how many meals you will need to eat away from home each week. For most people that would be lunch, 5 days a week plus let's say a Saturday night and one other weeknight for sport. That's 7 meals away from home that we have to prepare for.

Step 3: Calculate how many meals you are going to eat at home.

When you've worked out how many at home meals you are going to have, subtract that from the total to calculate how many meals you are going to eat at home. In this example, 21-7=14 meals at home.

Step 4: Simplify it. Variety may be the spice of life, but it leads to wishy-washy living and uncultured gluttony. So for us, we like to rotate the same 3 meals for breakfast every morning during the week. 7 more meals accounted for. That leaves 7 to decide on. 5 dinners and 2 lunches.

Step 5: Write it down. Put it all down on a piece of paper to see if you have any meal clashes.

Step 6: Add snacks. Think of one protein, one fat and one carb source that can be used for snacks that the kids can get themselves (or get from their lunchboxes) for each day. You can really simplify this by having the exact same snacks available every day.

Step 7: Decide what you are going to have and buy all your ingredients online.

For most people, planning a week's worth of food is exhausting. Most will give up even thinking about it and return to the Uni student lifestyle of "anything goes."

But if you're still with us, here's where the magic happens. Think about how much time each day you spend debating what to have for dinner. As soon as you schedule your food, you'll be absolutely amazed at how much more time and space you have in your brain.

The second benefit is that everybody stops asking you "what's for dinner."

Actually what we found to be the biggest time/energy killer is "what would you like for dinner?" In a family of 7 like ours that would mean 7 different meals, 42 times a week. A total of 294 meals!

Having a routine is the fundamental step you need to go through in order to have a successful life. Don't worry if you don't get it right first time, keep changing it where it fell apart - don't change a routine that is working.

Here's a sample one of ours.

	BREAKFAST	LUNCH	DINNER	AVAILABLE SNACKS
MONDAY	Egg Pies	Mango Salad + Cold Meat	Tacos	
	P: eggs	P: cold meat	P: beans + mince	P: Extra egg pies
	F: bacon+Avo	F: cold meat + grape seed oil dressing	F: avo + mince	F: trail mix
	CC: roasted pumpkin, spinach leaves	CC: salad greens	CC: lettuce shells + onions + capsicum + zucchini filling	C: melon
	SC: piece of fruit	SC: diced mango + strawberries	SC: salsa	

TUESDAY	Grain Free Granola	Fish Cakes & Salad	Fried Rice	
	P: natural yoghurt	P: fish	P: eggs + ham	P: ham slices
	F: seeds + nuts	F: fish + coconut oil	F: ham + coconut oil	F: banana bread
	CC: in seeds	CC: salad veg	CC: cauli-rice + veg + mushrooms	C: banana bread
	SC: banana + berries	SC: balsamic vinegar or lemon dressing	SC: HJ2 sorbet	
WEDNESDAY	Omelette	HJ1 Chicken nuggets	HJ1 Lasagne	
	P: eggs + cheese	P: chicken	P: mince	P: can of tuna
	F: cheese	F: coconut oil	F: mince	F: guacamole
	CC: diced veg + mushrooms	CC: shredded coconut	CC: carrots, mushroom, eggplant, cauli	C: carrot sticks
	SC: tomato	SC: tomato sauce	SC: tomato paste + tomato	
THURSDAY	Grain Free Granola	Lasagne Leftovers	Mini Pizzas	
	P: natural yoghurt		P: chicken breast base	P: cheese cubes
	F: seeds + nuts		F: cheese	F: cheese cubes
	CC: in seeds		CC: veg topping	C: fruit
	SC: banana + berries		SC: tomato paste	

FRIDAY	*Egg Pies*	*HJ2 Sushi*	*Spag Bol*	
	P: eggs	P: tuna	P: mince	P&F: Extra sushi
	F: bacon+Avo	F: avo	F: mince	C: fruit
	CC: roasted pumpkin, spinach leaves	CC: quinoa rice + cucumber + carrot	CC: spiralled zucchini	
	SC: piece of fruit	SC: piece fruit	SC: tomato puree	
SATURDAY	*Grain Free Granola*	*Garlic prawns*	*HJ2 sweet and sour pork*	
	P: natural yoghurt	P: prawns	P: pork	P: yoghurt
	F: seeds + nuts	F: coconut oil	F: coconut oil	F: yoghurt
	CC: in seeds	CC: salad vegetables	CC: quinoa rice + veg	C: fruit
	SC: banana + berries	SC: diced sweet potato	SC: pineapple	
SUNDAY	*Omelette*	*Chicken stirfry*	*Sunday Roast*	
	P: eggs + cheese	P: chicken	P: roast meat	P &F: Sesame seed butter (peanut butter)
	F: cheese	F: coconut oil + crushed seed mix	F: roast meat	
	CC: diced veg + mushrooms	CC: Veggies	CC: roast veg	C: Veggie sticks
	SC: tomato	SC: piece fruit	SC: pumpkin/ sweet potato	

P: protein

F: Fats

CC: Complex Carbs

SC: Simple Carbs

Measure your starting point

You never know if anything in your life is a success if you don't measure your starting point.

In the old days, explorers would draw a line in the sand with their boot and say, "I will never go back past that line again." It's time to draw your line in the sand.

Except your line will be on the wall.

A powerful memory for me (Julius) growing was after a swimming carnival I heard my mother talking to another mother about what had happened in the morning. My relay team had won our 4x100m freestyle race, but had come second in the medley relay. My mother's words were "we won the freestyle, but they lost the medley."

We won the freestyle, but *they* lost the medley. Seems insignificant to me as a grown man now, but to a young boy it hit home in a powerful way. People associate themselves with you when you win. But if you lose, they will subconsciously distance themselves from you.

I heard it a lot when I coached junior rugby teams - parents would say "*we* won" but never "*we* lost." It was always "*they* lost."

To a child, even if they don't consciously hear it and comprehend it, this type of thing, said without thought, is interpreted by their young mind as "If I lose (fail) I am not a part of the team/family."

Going back to the pencil in the wall - it is so important as a parent to be careful of what you say to your child. While we have to measure the starting point, while we have to draw a line in the sand, we have to do it in a way that empowers your child. We **DO NOT EVER** want them to feel like there is something wrong with them.

How do we avoid this?

We all measure ourselves. Mum, dad, kids, grandparent, everyone gets weighed and measured. Height, weight, tummy circumference, chest circumference, foot size, hand size. Measure a whole bunch of things and put them in a little notebook. To the child, you're doing it so that he/she can see how fast he/she is growing.

And they love it. So many times we'd catch Josh up against the wall, measuring himself and proudly telling us that he was getting taller.

Make sure you measure your child's weight, height and the waist circumference around the belly button. The result at this point is completely irrelevant and to compare them to a National Average is ridiculous.

Your child is not normal and not average. Your child is special and unique. Fuck the statisticians. Fuck the 'authorities,' fuck the school system and their 'reading age;' your child is perfect. And who'd want to be normal anyway. If you're reading this book, then you don't subscribe to the 'normal is good' philosophy.

Normal is average. Why celebrate average? Each of us is extraordinary in some way or another.

Draw that line in the sand. Because you and us, we're never coming back to this place again. The world needs to be put back on the rails, and we will do it alone if we have to - Sharny, Julius and you.

Drink way more water

We think every family should have an herb garden. Herbs are expensive to buy from the supermarket, but really, really easy to grow at home.

Quite often, when a child is thirsty, they feel it as hunger - keeping water levels up will reduce this one subconscious urge to snack all day.

But how do you do it - especially if kids are used to snacking, or used to drinking sweet drinks all day?

Well, for us it started in the herb garden. Our kids love the herb garden, they loved to see how everything grows each day (shallots grow about a centimetre every night) and they especially love watering the plants.

One weekend we went away, while we were away, we had a very hot spell and came back to wilted and limp herbs. Alexis and Danté noticed it immediately and asked me what had happened in the theatrical way kids do.

"Daddy, Daddy! Look at Basil, he's SICK!!"

I could have glossed over it, but it quickly struck me that here was a gift, a perfect learning opportunity for these kids, so I explained to them that the basil was sick, and that he was sick because we were away and couldn't give him a drink of water.

A few weeks later, Alexis (3) was complaining of having a sore head and feeling tired. While I was trying to work out what to do, I heard Danté (2) talking to her, as she laid on the couch.

"You no drink water Lecky? You sick? You wan' bottle?"

"Yeah Bud, get me some water... I'm limp."

It's moments like these where your heart feels like it is going to explode out of your chest with pride. I watched Danté fetch Alexis' water bottle and sit there with her making sure she drank it all. They sat there for a while talking about their water and how much they love water. Alexis even told Danté to drink his water so he wouldn't go limp too.

What amazes me to this day is that kids can find the right solution, because they look at life with uncomplicated eyes. If I get a headache, my first thought is "have we got any paracetamol?" Which is what I was doing while Danté was watering Alexis. I had thought of the cure, while the kids fixed the cause.

Give your kids a reason to have more water and they'll get it. For us, it was the herb garden. You may have better luck with pets. Kids know that pets only drink water; they don't drink anything else because it will make them sick. If you have pets, use this angle.

Also look at your own behaviour because kids copy their parents. If you're drinking soft drink and you're telling your kids to drink water, then to them you are a hypocrite. If you're feeling sick, ask your kids to get you a glass of water to make you feel better. They'll remember it for when they next get sick.

Swap your soft drink for water. Soft drink is not an adult's drink; it's a dangerous concoction of addictive chemicals. If you don't want your kids to drink it, don't have any in the house.

If you love the feel of soft drink or beer, just buy mineral water. We pour mineral water into a big glass of ice. Add a slice of lemon or lime and some mint leaves and you've got yourself a refreshing drink that your kids can share.

Our kids call mineral water "spicy water." They don't have it all the time, but if we make ourselves one, we make sure to have enough that we can share with the kids. It's just another way to keep up with their water needs.

Water should be readily accessible all the time. Kids will drink water if it's in front of them, but will not actively seek it out unless they are really thirsty. Make sure your kids have easy access to water, and that you offer it to them all the time too. Have a bottle for each child in the fridge door that they can get themselves. At mealtime, this bottle should sit next to their plate.

Eat carbohydrates, fats and proteins at every meal

"Balanced diet."

You don't hear those words too much any more. Before this obesity epidemic, parents used to say that the key to a healthy life was to eat a balanced diet. We haven't heard that since we were kids, partly because nobody makes money promoting a balanced diet, and more realistically, the meaning of a balanced diet has changed.

Back in the early 80's a balanced diet was meat, veggies, fruit, vegetables and some starch to keep us going. Back in the 80's we lived a largely outdoor lifestyle, so the starch, which most people nowadays call "carbs" was necessary.

We'll talk about carbs, fats and proteins in the next sections, but what is most important is that to be at their physical and mental peak, children need a balance of each.

Carbs, fats and proteins are collectively called macronutrients. Macros for short. And here's the key point. Everybody's macronutrient balance is as unique as his or her fingerprint.

What your child's body needs depends on what they do with it. For example, a desk bound secretary is going to have a completely different macro balance to her 8 year old son, who loves swimming and reading.

That's pretty obvious though, so let's say the secretary shares her desk with another secretary of the same age, height and weight. I can tell you from experience, 99% of the time, secretary 1 and secretary 2 will have different macronutrient needs.

Because what a body needs, takes into account so many variables

Here's a list, and it's not exhaustive:

- Genetics
- Environment
- Age
- Previous 3 months of intake
- Injuries
- Illness
- Personality
- Stress levels
- Sleeping patterns
- Exercise
- Meal timing
- Volume of food consumed
- Hydration

- Tiredness
- Fitness level
- The amount of work the brain has to do compared to normal
- What is being eaten
- Stimulants or relaxants
- Outside temperature
- Bedroom temperature
- Type of clothes
- Etc.

We know a doctor, who can work this all out for you, but he charges $400 per hour and needs a minimum of 12 hours of time with you to calculate your macronutrient needs *at a given moment in time.*

Macronutrient needs change from day to day and hour to hour. So the only realistic way to work it out is by yourself through iterative trial and error.

To work it out your child's macronutrient needs, you have to start somewhere. Where that is does not matter at all, just like your child's initial height and weight; it is just a benchmark to work from.

The first thing to do is track what you and your family consume on a day-to-day basis. Keeping track for just one week will give you a huge insight into your eating habits. More importantly, it will give you a starting point. A reference point.

Let us introduce you to an app called *MyFitnessPal.*

MyFitnessPal is phenomenal and the creators of it deserve a Nobel Prize. It makes the job of counting calories and macros completely idiot proof, and it is free!

All you do is input your foods that you eat, and the app will look through it's library of foods to find out how much of each macronutrient you've consumed, as well as the calories and a bunch of other useful stuff. If you eat anything that has a barcode, you just scan the barcode and it will input all the info automatically.

At the end of each day, *MyFitnessPal* will tell you how many calories you consumed (important) as well show you as a pie chart that tells you how much of each macro you've eaten (far more important).

Until this app was created, calculating macros and calories was tedious, mind numbing work. Now, we recommend everybody use it in the same way that having a budgeting app helps to keep spending under control.

But here's the even better part.

Since you're now doing your shopping online, you'll be able to calculate your macronutrients in advance and tweak it for what you would like to have!

Close Mum's Restaurant

Realistically, how do you implement this new way of eating?

We wouldn't try to control the macros in the first week; we'd just measure them. You've got enough of a job on your hands getting an entire family to fit into your new routine, as well as making sure everybody eats the same meal.

If your first week is anything like ours, you'll be flat out helping your family adjust to eating together, and more importantly eating the same meal. You are not a restaurant where people can order whatever they want.

If you find yourself, like us, cooking a different dinner for each person in the family, stop that shit right bloody now! You're no slave. You're the parent and for the next week, "we eat what mummy or daddy cooks. That's it."

A missed meal won't hurt a child. They will push you, mentally trick you or emotionally blackmail you, but if you keep your cool and don't buckle to their tantrums, you'll find the process happens so much faster.

If your toddler throws a tantrum and refuses to eat their food, don't get angry, just turn around and walk away. Seriously, it is the most amazing thing - we read it in a book and tried it. It sounds too good to be true, but when the toddler is misbehaving, we turn around and walk away. In less than 5 minutes, the tantrum has stopped and they say sorry. Truly a miracle.

Spend the first week freeing yourself of *Mum's Restaurant*. If you like, track your own macros for the week. Kids do have an off switch, unlike us adults. When they are full, they won't eat any more. Children are actually better at controlling their macros than we are.

Because kids leave a bit on their plate or the floor, tracking what they ate is going to be a lot harder than tracking what you ate. Just make sure you are eating the same meal with the same macronutrient balance. Theirs will just be a different sized plate, but the proportions of each ingredient should still be the same as yours.

This is why it is so important that everybody eats the same meal.

If you don't track the macros for the first week, do it on the second. Remember that having fit, healthy, happy kids is a lifelong journey - it's not a quick fix and forget, it's not a race. Don't overwhelm yourself with trying to change everything at once.

Little gentle nudges back onto the path of health are much easier and harder to detect than huge shifts. People don't like to change too much at once, so taking longer is better than taking less time. If it takes you a month to get everyone to eat the same, good for you - that's faster than it took us!

Find balance first, before you tinker

You've finally got the whole family eating the same thing each meal and your routine is more or less fixed and predictable each week. You've measured your macros for at least one week.

Scroll back through your week to find imbalanced meals. Put a red mark next to the meal and fix it for next week. Have a look at the following diagram to see what an imbalanced meal looks like.

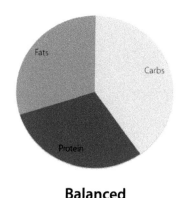

Balanced

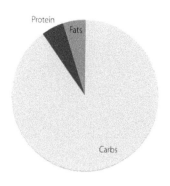

Imbalanced

Remember that you are balancing the pie chart for calories, not for weight. Having a meal that is balanced by weight is going to make you sick, and if you can actually stomach it, make you very fat.

Because fats are very high in calories, you won't need as much of them on your plate as say, complex carbs; which are low in calories.

Just by tracking your intake for one week, you will have become aware. You will forever look at your food and be able to kind of guesstimate what it is missing.

You see, the thing most people are getting wrong is not that they eat too much, but that they either eat too much of one macro, or don't eat enough of another. Now that you have your routine and your benchmark, just scroll through last week and make sure you have some of each macro in every single meal from now on. That's it.

Strategic snacking

Many Aussie families are used to eating 3 meals and 3 snacks a day. If your kids aren't in the habit of having snacks, then we strongly recommend just trying to give them only balanced meals.

Let us explain.

Once your children wake up, feed them a balanced breakfast immediately. Try to make sure they are full before leaving the table to brush their teeth and go on about their morning. To make sure they are full, remove potential distractions and make sure that breakfast is at the same time and place every single day.

Now, wait until they start showing the signs of being hungry, but make sure it is hungry, not thirsty by keeping up their water intake. Once they are hungry, expose them another balanced plate and see what they eat.

If they eat all of it, then you've hit their macro sweet spot for that meal. All you do then, is adjust their meal times next week to catch them as they are feeling hungry. Many children will not be able to only eat 3 times a day, in which case you'll just need to adjust their meal times accordingly.

If they are hungry only an hour or so after eating breakfast, you may need to increase the fat content of their breakfast. This is the start of finding the macro sweet spot. We'll go into more of these triggers in each of the individual macro chapters.

If they ate a little of everything, that's great. Often though, your child will only eat one type of food in their snack, usually a carbohydrate. This too is alright, only if they have been playing all morning.

It means that they are burning off their food energy nice and fast. Giving them a snack of fruit will encourage them to keep playing until lunchtime, which should be a sit down, balanced plate.

As long as breakfast, lunch and dinner are balanced, it is alright for kids to top their energy up with a small amount of sugary carbs to keep them going until the next meal. Don't fall into the trap of giving them biscuits, breads or other starches as a snack though; the body can only store a very small amount of sugar.

If kids are hungry for something, they will seek it out. The key is for you as their parent to be aware. As we said before, children have a much better thermostat than we do. As long as they are exposed to a balanced plate at every main meal, they will choose what their bodies need.

This is so fundamentally important that we are going to put it into it's own section right here:

They already know

Children are much better equipped than we are for making food choices. Young children are yet to be exposed to the seduction of food marketers, or the addictive substances laced in the food we adults have become accustomed to.

Children know. They already know. You just have to provide them with the selection, and because they are still so in tune with their bodies, they will intuitively consume a balanced diet.

And you know what's awesome too?

You were a kid once, and not that long ago - so you just have to unlearn all the bullshit you've been sold and you too will be able to listen to your body. We're sure by now you'll be noticing how your attitude toward food is so entrenched in behaviour implanted without you knowing.

Like dessert.

People haven't always had dessert. It's not a staple; it's not even necessary and not good for you. Dessert companies suggested it and marketed it, and now because we've always done it, we continue to do it.

But you're starting to feel different, because after eating a balanced diet, you'll notice your "needs" for certain foods are not as powerful any more. The strings that the marketers are playing aren't that seductive any more. It's because your body is properly fed.

You are becoming an intuitive eater, just like your amazing kids.

Can you see the MASSIVE distinction? Intuitive feels the same as reactive. But instead of eating what you want to taste, you are now eating *what your body needs to be fuelled by* - and it's happening without you even trying...

How cool is that!

Carbohydrate

In the next few chapters, we are going to discuss the 3 macronutrients. Proteins, carbohydrates and fats. Let's start with the very misunderstood carbohydrate.

Technically speaking a carbohydrate is any combination of sugar molecules. It is our body's most easily accessible source of fuel. Not only do we need carbohydrates to physically function at our peak, but our brains actually use carbohydrates as fuel. This is why kids get so hungry for sugar when they are learning something new.

Imagine a carbohydrate molecule as a grain of sand that you are trying to wash down the sink. The grain of sand in its simple form is easy to wash down the sink. Just like sugars, we can wash a whole lot of sand down the sink very fast. Sugars are like grains of sand.

Mud is a little harder to wash down than sand, but with a bit of work it can go down much easier. Mud can, however clog the pipes. Starchy carbohydrates are like mud. They are easily digested, but can clog up very easily. Examples of starches include potatoes, breads and pastas. Both sugars and starchy carbohydrates are called simple carbohydrates.

Now, lets say that the grains of sand are all joined together to make stones. Stones can still fit down the drain pipe if we break them down into sand, which isn't that hard - but it takes energy and you will find it hard to clog the system because you can't really break them down fast enough. Vegetables are like stones. Vegetables are called complex carbohydrates.

Stones that cannot be broken down into sand, but can still be pushed down the drain, can be used to clear the drain of any gunk left in the pipes, from the mud or from the animal fats that we have washed down there. Stones that cannot be broken down into sand are what we call fibre, fibre is so complex a carbohydrate that it basically passes through the body unchanged, or undigested.

Never restrict carbohydrates from children

We're sure you've heard about "low carb" eating. "Low carb" eating has been misunderstood and resultantly misguided people for the last 20 years. As we said before, people have this misconception that the only carbs there are, are starches.

We know a lot of people who have done low carb diets and are still doing their low carb diets after many years, Their bodies have unfortunately adapted and as a result, they can only eat the tiniest portions while remaining overweight. These poor people are always sick and depressed because they just cannot control their binge eating, and they get very few micronutrients needed for survival.

And these are adults. Please, for the sake of your kids, never ever restrict carbs, or any macronutrient for that matter.

Balance carbohydrate types

Just like the three macronutrients, children need a balance of carbohydrates. It's no good giving them only vegetables, just like it is no good giving them only fruits.

We find it best to ensure that every meal has more complex carbohydrates than simple carbohydrates. If children are particularly active, we will add starchy carbohydrates.

For example, an 8-year-old boy is playing a game of sport at 9am. For breakfast at 7am, we would make sure for his carbs, he has some vegetables as well as starch, finished off with a piece of fruit. A great meal for this would be fried fish patties.

Essentially you just steam a bunch of veggies (complex carbs) and some potato (starch), and then quickly blend them with some fish (protein). Form into patties and fry in some coconut oil (fat). After your son has eaten his fill of fish cakes, give him some melon (simple carbohydrate).

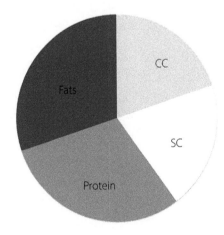

Pie chart showing balanced carbs
(SC = simple carbs *and* starchy carbs)

We would always offer fruit *after* the meal, so that they already have some vegetables in the system. It doesn't work the other way around. Imagine trying to eat a piece of broccoli after having fruit salad... probably not going to happen.

About 15 or so minutes before the game, we'd offer him some banana (simple carbs) dipped in peanut butter (fat and protein). As we said before, he may not want the peanut butter, but he'll want them after the game; once he is rehydrated.

See the *Reader Questions* at the back of this book for a great rehydration recipe to use instead of Gatorade or PowerAde. If your child is playing sport at school, you can substitute sesame seed butter for peanut butter. Check your *Healthy Junk 1* for that recipe.

Let's get back to balancing your carbohydrates, if you have an overweight child, a great place to help them lose the bloat without them knowing, is to just stop giving them starchy carbohydrates for a while. If your child is hyperactive, skinny and always hungry, the opposite is recommended; increase their starches.

In both cases remember that your carbohydrates still need to balance out your proteins and fats. If your child is used to eating starchy carbs and you take them off the plate, you have to replace them with a balance of simple and complex carbohydrates.

The final point here is that you should try to make sure that while starting out, complex carbohydrates (vegetables) form the bulk of every meal. Complex carbs will take a lot of space on your plate, but will not take much space on the macro pie chart though.

Remember that the end goal is to balance your macros. The pie chart then, looks very different to the plate. So when we say to make complex carbohydrates the bulk, it is because most children have a micronutrient deficiency, from years of eating too few vegetables. Increase their vegetables so that they top up their depleted stores.

White powders are dangerous

While we are on the subject of carbohydrates, we have a general rule of thumb that works really well for us and the families that we have helped. Eliminate white powders from your life.

Unfortunately, refined white sugar, refined flour and all product made with them are just way too high in carbohydrates to be even possible to match with proteins and fats. Refined white powders are highly addictive and are part of the reason that our "balance thermostat" is just off - our bodies just want to overdose on simple white powders. Simple white powders carry none of the micronutrient nutrition that fruits carry, remember before how we said that carbohydrates carry more than just energy, well white powders carry only energy, something our primitive bodies just cannot get a control over.

So if your family is used to eating bread, pasta, pizzas and breakfast cereal, you'll want to look at replacing those ingredients for safer alternatives. For ideas on how to do this, we created our cookbook called *Healthy Junk*. In it you will find recipes for over 100 different junk foods, made with healthy ingredients.

We will help you out with a couple of very easy white powder replacements right now though.

- If you love pasta or spaghetti as we do, simply spiral some zucchini and boil for about a minute - you won't be able to taste any difference.

- If you like pizza, replace the dough with a thinly sliced chicken breast - once again, you will not taste any difference.

- Rice is not really a white powder, but is a starch that can be overused in modern cooking, so we replace ours with a quickly blended cauliflower. Boil the cauliflower rice for much less time than real rice and your kids will never notice the difference.

In one of the later chapters, we will delve into the potential dangers of sugars and wheat. Both of which have received a lot of adverse attention as the world tries to discover a cure for obesity. In the meantime, lets look at our next macronutrient, fat.

Fat

A diet without fat is like a campfire fuelled only by tissues.

In our book *Never Diet Again*, we dive quite deeply into fats and the types of fats, but rather than make this a science lesson out of a text book, we'll discuss why fat is important, and why it is dangerous to exclude it from a child's diet.

Fats are an essential part of a balanced diet. How do we know this? Because for the last 20 years we have lived in a *low fat* obsessed world. Fat is an energy source, just like carbohydrates. It's just that each molecule of fat carries 3 times as many calories than carbs.

If you eat fat, nearly all of it gets used. If you eat a natural carbohydrate (fruit or vegetable), not all of it is used for fuel. Can you see how it is quite easy to blame fat for the obesity epidemic? Cut out all the fat in your diet and you won't get fat?

Wrong.

Fortunately for us, fat is not only tasty, but is actually very important to our cells and endocrine system (hormones). Hormones control so many vital functions in the body, functions that are even more important in growing children. Hormones control growth. Hormones control puberty, hormones control appetite, hormones control mood.

Fats play two vital roles when it comes to hormones. Firstly, hormones are carried around on cholesterol, something else that has gotten a bad rap. Cholesterol is made in the body by combining a fat and a protein molecule. Hormones ride cholesterol like postmen ride bikes. Without the bike, the message is delayed or not delivered.

The second vital role is that fats kind of mop up the excess hormones. So you don't get a hormone overdose. A good example for this is when mum gets her period once a month, her hormones overdrive. If mum is eating a low fat diet, she will feel this at a much higher frequency than if she had been eating a balanced diet with fats included.

Before we continue with beating the "fat is good" drum, it is important for you to understand that fat is good as part of a *balanced* diet. Some people have swung right across the other way and now only eat a high fat, low carb diet. Just like a low fat diet, this will eventually lead to problems.

Too much fat, just like too much carbohydrate will make your children off balance, which will propagate as weight gain, mood swings, stress or illness. It's up to you to manage how much fat they intake, but as long as they are eating the right kind of fats, the volume they can consume is very likely much higher than you think.

The state of the obesity epidemic alone should convince you to ignore the 'fat free' aisle and rethink your fat intake. But before you go cooking up a meal of just pork crackling, there are some things you need to know about fats.

Firstly, as a general rule, if you're going to cook with fat, only cook with saturated fats. Saturated fats are solid at room temperature. Saturated fats are what we call heat stable, they don't change composition at higher temperatures. Unsaturated fats do.

Animal fats, butterfat (like ghee) and coconut oil are high in saturated fats.

We use extra virgin, cold pressed coconut oil for most of our cooking needs. Coconut oil, unlike animal fat, requires less processing to make, and with animal fats, you have to trust that the animal was raised unstressed and grass fed without disease or drugs.

Coconut oil is easily digested and put to use by the body. It is a medium chain fatty acid, therefore used in the body much like a sugar, except without the insulin spike. Being a medium chain fat, coconut oil is actually very good for your child's immune system. It is a disease fighter!

As a general rule, the shorter the chain, the better at fighting disease. Mother's breastmilk has very short chain fats, and is why breastfed babies can stay healthy even when the whole family has the flu.

That's why Sharny and I have so many kids. While she is breastfeeding, we all take turns on her boob so we don't get sick.

I'm just joking to see if you're still with me. We drink cows milk, because it's so much more natural to breastfeed from a cow.

Fats are essential for protecting your body from disease. Saturated fats are essential to building strong cell walls. Unsaturated fats are important for reducing inflammation and for reducing bad cholesterol. All natural fats are good for you and your children, so wouldn't it make sense to include them in a balanced diet?

Fats are a very interesting subject that we could write an entire dissertation on, but the overwhelming truth is that your children need them in order to grow up unhindered by food issues. Just like it is important to balance the macronutrients, it is just as important to balance the fats.

Too much of one type of fat can be bad for you, just like too little of one type of fat can be bad for you. Unlike carbohydrates though, it is quite hard to overeat on fats - they just make you feel sick.

Here are the rules we live by when it comes to fat.

Only eat natural fats

Trans fats are created when a polyunsaturated fat is blasted with hydrogen to make it solid at room temp. Margarine is not natural and will kill you. We tipped a tub of margarine in the garden of our gym once, 6 months later it was still there - ants wouldn't even eat it.

One of our clients owned a funeral home and he said that you could tell when someone had been a margarine eater because the pan that they cremate them in would come out with the remains as well as a layer of what seemed like plastic on the pan.

Only cook with saturated fats

Unsaturated fats are unstable at high temperatures and can become carcinogenic. Unsaturated fats are still important though so we use our unsaturated fats in salad dressings. Examples of oils that we do not cook with include grape seed oil, sesame oil, flaxseed (linseed) oil, avocado oil and olive oil (not as bad).

To tell saturated fats are solid at room temp, and can be used in cooking.

Unsaturated fats are liquids and can't be used in cooking. If a fat (other than coconut) is solid, but the ingredients say it's plant oil, stay well clear – this is a Trans fat.

Only buy extra virgin, cold pressed plant oils

You may be buying the right oil, and not cooking with it, but the manufacturer could have compromised it when they made it. Ensure that it was cold pressed, and that it has not been chemically tampered with. Cheap oils almost always are bleached or chemically extracted. Steer well clear of human intervention.

Eat oily fish

Oily fish contain fantastic anti-inflammatory properties and are not as easily tampered with the way land animals can be.

Eat fats to stop hunger

Fats help with the feeling of fullness. We don't cut the fat off our cuts of meat, unless our meal is already skewed towards being higher in fat. A roast is a great example of a time when we trim off visible fat - most roast cuts are very high in fats without the layer of fat around the outside too.

Balance fats and carbs

Fats and carbs provide us with energy; use your *MyFitnessPal* pie chart to balance them. Because fat has a much higher calorie density, you'll need a lot less of it than your carbs. Balance the pie chart, not the space on your plate.

Avocado and fish are our best friends

You may find the hardest thing to balance is your unsaturated fats, I mean, you can't cook with them and kids won't eat a salad at every meal, so blend up some guacamole and serve with a piece of fish to get a good dose of unsaturated fats if you find that dinner has come and they haven't had any unsaturated fats today. Also check your chocolate mousse recipe in *Healthy Junk 1*, it is made with avocado.

Be sensible

You know when you're eating too much fat. The only time you aren't is if you buy packaged food, or eat out. If you cook most of your meals at home, you control the balance. As we said before, if you don't have a plan for your family's eating, you will be at the mercy of someone else's. Food is a competitive industry. The most profitable food companies create repeat buyers, so it makes sense for them to make food that is addictive.

Protein

After reading the carb and fat section, we need to reiterate that *imbalance* is what causes kids to seek balance. If they don't find a certain fat in their diet, they will just keep eating what's in front of you until they find it.

Protein plays this game perfectly. Your body craves protein like it craves water. Proteins are the building blocks of the body. Think of them like bricks. All of your internal and external structure needs these bricks to support you, to support life.

After the Vietnam War, the UN tried to find out why so many kids were malnourished, why they were sick and dying. Part of their study found that some families had much healthier kids than the rest. The only reason was that the mothers of these families had been crushing prawns into their children's rice. It was this added protein that made them healthier, even in the face of Agent Orange.

But let's maybe look at it differently. Without protein in a child's diet, they will be incapable of growing the way nature intended. They will be malnourished. In Vietnam, these kids couldn't find the protein. In our time, kids have access to unlimited food. They WILL continue eating to find the nourishment that they need.

Protein is essential to a child's development. But you already knew that. Where you may differ from another reader is whether you like to eat animals or not. Our family goes through phases of eating animal meat for a few weeks and then sometimes we'll go without animal meat for a month or two.

We don't do this for any other reason than because it feels right.

In our family, we have come to the conclusion that we need meat, but not nearly as much as we thought we did. Once again, we come back to balance. To balance our protein needs, we try to get protein from many different sources. It is hard to mix proteins in each meal, so we try to balance our protein over the week, or the month.

One thing we have discovered in our family, and you may or may not be the same, is that we feel better and perform better if we eat less red meat. I love red meat; I come from South Africa where we used to eat slabs of beef straight off the braai (BBQ). But something has happened, maybe I've changed or the beef has changed, but I can't eat too much of it without feeling tired and a little queasy in the stomach.

We have found a difference in organic grass fed beef, but not a huge amount. Pork makes all of us ill, even if we get our pork from Sharny's dad, who has his own pastured pigs who eat only good quality food scraps.

The only conclusion I can come to is that when you are all eating a balanced diet, your body gets used to it and expects it. Overeating on something to the detriment of something else puts you out of balance. If I eat a massive piece of steak, I feel like I need to balance it out over the next few meals with lots of vegetables. The kids are the same.

This to me means that the concept of balance is a driver from inside; our kids are not tampered with unrealistic food expectations like "finish what's on your plate", and are not exposed to chemical, addictive foods. As a result, we just give them options at every meal and their bodies will tell them what they need or don't need.

Once you get to this point, you can actually predict what they are going to eat, in order to reduce wastage.

When your child's body is in balance, and you present them with options, they will choose what their body needs. Like everything in nature, the human body likes to stay in balance. Scientists call this homeostasis.

Tinkering with your balance

Now that you know a little about each of the macros, you should have a go at putting it all together.

The place to be looking is not at your plate, but at your *MyFitnessPal* pie chart. What proportions of each macronutrient have you been eating? *What ratio we've been hitting*, we say.

It doesn't matter where you start, by now you should have an idea of what that pie chart looks like. There are a few opinions on what is a good macro ratio, but they are just that - opinions. We'd suggest starting with a popular one of them and then tinkering to find your perfect formula.

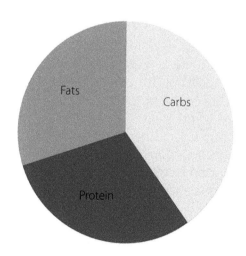

For young children, a great place to start is 40% carbs, 30% fats and 30% protein. This is a goal, it is a ratio to be mindful of while you plan your meals and more importantly when you debrief the day or week. It is not a rule.

As we said right in the beginning chapter, the only way to find out your macro sweet spot, it through trial and error. This is where your routine becomes absolutely essential. You will never know if your child's behaviour is a result of their food, if you have no basis for comparison.

By now, you would have been in a routine long enough that you can observe changes in your children's behaviour. These are signs to look for when tinkering with their balance.

As long as you have stuck to your routine, anything out of the ordinary should raise a nutritional flag. It has been far easier to blame something outside of our control when a child changes behaviour or falls ill. Doing so would make you rely on outside help. You don't need to do that any more.

But think of it this way, if your child develops a snotty nose for example. We normally say that there is a cold going around. Wouldn't it make sense first to check their last 3 meals as well as their hydration before looking at the day care centre or school?

The gut lining is designed to let things in, absorb them. The skin, nose and mouth are designed to keep stuff out. We are far more exposed to internal nutritional imbalance than we are to bugs from outside.

So that's what we'd do. First, mentally roll back time to see if the child has had enough water. Secondly, check if they have eaten anything new in the past 3 meals that may indicate an intolerance or allergy. If no to both, check that for other signs, i.e. only ate the fruit, or stuffed himself or herself full of chicken.

All of the following signs can point us to a cause.

Tiredness:

Usually a sign of too much high calorie starch or sugar in the last meal, roll back the sugars and carbs in the next meal.

Irritability or excitability:

Usually a sign of too much simple carbohydrate. Kids are very in tune with food, so in just the same way that we can go a little crazy on an energy drink, they too can go crazy on sugars/fruit. Good idea to give them lots of water and get them outside for a play.

Refusing food normally eaten:

Usually a sign that somewhere in the last few meals they ate too much of one macro, or ate something that disagreed with their body. Offer water and monitor their progress. Should be back to balance in one day.

Eating more than normal:

Either a sign that there is too much sugar in the meal, or that they have just been super active before eating. Remember that the brain uses a lot of sugar to run, so they could be burning up fuel even by doing nothing.

We give our kids fruit last in each meal, because if we give it to them first, insulin kicks in and turns them into uncontrollable feeding machines. The opposite is true if your child doesn't eat much at all - give them fruit first to pick up their appetite.

Being hungry soon after a meal:

Usually a sign that there was either too much simple carbohydrate or not enough fat in the last meal.

Illness:

Look for anomalies in eating before looking to the doctor for an explanation and a packet of pills. Give plenty of water.

Sudden changes in behaviour:

Check that the last food eaten did not contain additives. Additives are chemicals we know very little about, and can wreak havoc in a small child's body. This is why we refuse to buy packaged food.

Another cause can be dehydration, a small glass of water adds up to quite a large percentage of the child's body size, so missing one can be similar to an adult not drinking for a whole week.

Eating only one food group:

Not normally a cause for concern unless it goes on for longer than 3 days. Usually the kids need a particular food group more than the others in times of growth. If there is a more sinister issue, it will also propagate in one of the other ways listed.

Saying things out of character:

If they are rude or obnoxious, check for additives, dehydration or macro imbalance. If the behaviour is good behaviour, i.e. your child has suddenly become FAR more mature and easy to get along with, examine in depth the last meal. It may be their macro sweet spot.

Hay fever, bloating in the stomach, going to the toilet often, itchiness or hives:

A sign of food intolerance, check for new ingredients that have been introduced in the past day. Common causes could be wheat, dairy, nuts, shellfish or additives.

Laziness or quietness:

Usually a sign of too much fat or too much starchy carbohydrates. Let the child sleep and make the next meal have less fat/starchy carbs (more veggies).

Sleeplessness:

Too much water before bed or too much starchy carbohydrate before bed. Also check for additives in their dinner.

Excessive thirst:

Usually a sign that the child has eaten a lot of carbohydrate, not usually a concern but be mindful of other behavioural changes. Give lots of water.

Inflammation in the face / red eyes:

This is a sure sign of a food allergy or intolerance. Pay close attention to your child, if they struggle with breathing as well, call an ambulance.

Rapid weight gain or rapid weight loss:

This is a major cause for concern. Not in the first few weeks of your routine, as their bodies find their balance and rid themselves of toxins by becoming inflamed and then very quickly, almost overnight dropping the bloat. If you have been keeping up with your routine for a while now, try to find out what is causing the rapid weight loss or gain, clues will be found in their food.

Some of the above issues can happen instantly, others can be quite gradual. If you give your child a balanced plate, they will balanced their own diet and will generally not overeat; as long as they don't have the archaic mindset of "finish everything on your plate."

But, there are signs that you may need to tinker with their weekly/daily macro ratio.

If they are always hungry, try reducing their simple carbohydrates and replacing them with saturated fats.

Too much protein makes a smelly child. Excess protein is sweated our breathed out of the system and can make your kid really stink. If your child smells like Grandpas breath, just reduce the overall protein, whilst simultaneously increasing carbs, but not starches.

Too little protein propagates as lethargy or weakness. Paleness is another sure sign that the protein needs of your little one aren't being met.

Too much complex carbohydrate will give them a sore tummy and clog them up with barbed wire poo; **too little complex carbohydrate** will make them not poo enough.

Too much fat and they will get a greasy skin, or their poo will leave a waxy layer on top of the water. **Too little fat** and their attention span can be very short. Please check this before you go down the path of pharmaceuticals.

A smelly wee is a sure sign that your child is **dehydrated.** Give them water before their dehydration changes their mental state too!

You'll be able to find out how your kids are reacting to food and with a little detective work, understand why. You've had decades of eating experience more than them, so think back through your life for potential solutions.

To recap, start with a ratio of around 40:30:30 carbs:fat:protein and tinker from there based on your observations. Observe acute (fast, precise) changes in behaviour as well as chronic (long lasting). Adjust their macros accordingly.

Nutrient dense, not calorie dense

Now that you've been using *MyFitnessPal* for a little time, you've no doubt wondered why there is such a big difference in the weight of a food, and the weight of the macronutrients in the food. For example, 100g or grapes, we would assume would provide 100g of carbohydrates, but it only provides 17 grams.

What happens to the rest of the grape? What *is* the rest of it?

The bulk is actually water weight and fibre, but that's not all. Both are obviously important, but what are more important for this chapter are the *micro*nutrients that come in with the macronutrients. Things you know you need, like vitamins and minerals, antioxidants and acids.

Most people just look at macros and try to hit a macro goal each day and leave it at that. But that leaves the door open to *pure* energy sources. Pure energy sources carry no macronutrients. We say that they have no nutrition. Think about your body like your home. Pure energy is like only ever bringing food into the house.

A home needs so much more than just food, it needs cleaning products, telephones, internet, power, toilet paper, shampoo, clothes for the occupants, the list goes on.

Your body is the same, and for a growing child this is even more important; there is so much more to performing at your physical peak than protein, carbs, fats and water. They may be essentials to survive, but to truly flourish, a body needs micronutrients - the more the better.

We thought about going into what micronutrients do and what to look for and how to eat them, but we've actually got a very simple formula for making sure you get adequate micros.

The study of micronutrients is like studying the stars, you can stare at them for a lifetime and the more you learn the more you realise you don't know. It can be quite overwhelming, but fear not - we don't really need to know anything about micros, because with our little formula, your kids will be getting 99% of their micros easily.

Once you've got this, anything that you or your kids might be missing will be fixed with the odd craving here and there or pinch of Himalayan rock salt once in a while. Here goes.

"Cook everything yourself and serve on a balanced plate with a variety of colours, from natural ingredients raised naturally and your micros will take care of themselves."

To make processed foods, manufacturers essentially strip out the intricate, natural micronutrients that are *good for your children*, and replace them with cheap chemical micronutrients *that are good for the manufacturers profit.*

Avoid processed foods as much as possible to get as many of the natural micros as you can, that's why we recommend cooking everything yourself. If you're eating a balanced macro diet, using only natural ingredients raised naturally, then you and your family are consuming the best possible ingredients you can, the only added thought then is to have a variety of colours.

Each vegetable and fruit, and even each type of fat, has different micronutrients in them. Eating as much colour variety as possible will help to spread the micronutrient load and essentially allow your children's bodies to pick and choose what they need.

If you and your family are used to eating only packaged processed foods, then the process of *balancing your plate* then *increasing the nutrient density* will feel like walking out of a dark cave into a bright sunny day.

Once you graduate past the calorie/macro model to the wellness model, you will see that food is so much more than how much body fat your kids have.

Food is life, food is vitality, food is energy!

Going from packaged foods, to organic natural produce can be quite a steep learning curve and for the first month at least it can be much more expensive. Your body and your children's bodies will be lapping up all the amazing micronutrients that they are missing, and will appear to be eating constantly.

But don't fear, the body is a wonderful gift, with the capacity to self regulate. Once they have replenished what they need, and once they have rid themselves of the toxins put there by processed foods, the food bill drops dramatically. They simply don't need as much.

You'll also notice that they don't quarrel as much, they don't need sleep as much (neither will you) and they certainly don't have that vacuous lust for something more in their lives, because when you fuel yourself correctly, when your children fuel themselves correctly, life truly becomes an adventure from the inside out.

So many people right now are searching desperately for their purpose. But I tell you, once you fuel correctly; you will find that no amount of outside searching will bring you to your purpose. You'll be delighted and shocked to find that your purpose is simply to be you and to live the life set out for you.

Be the best version of you that you can be.

Everything boils down to your internal environment. We call it, this collection of macronutrient balancing and micronutrient balancing the art of nutrition. If you only ever consider calories, you're missing the point of life.

Potential poisons

Before we go into wheat, sugar, dairy, soy and all the current 'trend diets,' please remember that when someone tells you to cut a food out of your diet, do your own research first. If it sounds ridiculous, like cutting out fruit, then it probably is.

So without further ado, we'll go through the pros and cons of each of the current 'trendy foods to stay away from'

First and foremost, let's check in on sugar.

Sugar

People have such a pitchfork rage against sugar, and I'll tell you the science behind why. As I said before, sugar is a simple carbohydrate. All carbohydrates are made up of sugar molecules. The problem we have, according to the science buffs is that fructose, the sugar found in fruit, is very easily turned into fat. When fructose is abused, it can cause liver damage. Fructose is more addictive than heroin. Fructose is therefore to blame for obesity.

Sounds logical, and in the right context it is. We'll play devils advocate for a minute and run this by you again. Fructose is the sugar in fruit and we've been eating fruit for millions of years. We've only ever had an obesity epidemic in the last 20 or 30 years though. If fruit made us fat, then surely we would have had an obesity epidemic as long as fruit has been around?

Part of the marketing for the anti-sugar people is to educate us on how low fat diets are bad. Which we've already discussed are.

The anti-sugar people decided that it's best to cut out all sugar, replacing it with fat. We are Willing to bet that in a few years time, the gurus will *discover* that sugar is actually essential to life, and the diet media will then say, "If it's not fat, and it's not sugar, then it must be protein."

For years we'll have people quit protein. This lack of protein will cause people to go gaunt and sick and the diet media will then turn against something else, like water.

If we go back through the research, and even to Robert Lustig's now famous speech on sugar, we see that while fructose does indeed get converted into fat by the liver, he still says that we need to eat fruit.

Here's the deal; *too much sugar* is the enemy. And that is it.

Too much sugar is the enemy. Just like too much of anything is the enemy. 20 years ago, someone must have said, "Too much fat in your diet will make you gain weight." We went through a revolution and changed it to "fat makes you fat."

Don't believe in sensationalism. Sugar is important in your diet. Too much sugar will cause obesity and will cause liver damage. The real problem is not fruit, but added sugar.

Fruit is *nutrient* dense, where foods with added sugar are generally *calorie* dense, nutrient poor.

What do we recommend? Don't buy processed crap, because manufacturers know sugar is addictive, so they hide it in nearly everything.

Remember that food manufacturers make money off repeat customers, so will lure your children in with bright colours and animal pictures, lure *you* in with a large "low fat" sticker, and hook you both with a ton of added refined sugar.

Don't limit your child's fruit intake. Fruit carries with it some of our most important micronutrients - if your kids don't get them, they will search for them in other sweet tasting foods.

Finally, kids are very different to adults. You, as an adult, may in fact be abusing sugar. Years or overeating sugar, via added sugars and high fructose corn syrup, has given you a high level of insulin in your body, which is linked to nearly every degenerative disease known to man.

But it takes time to get to this point. No child needs to go on a fruit free diet. Just like no child should be eating processed sugar or refined sugar anyway. Refined sugars are no longer sugars though, and should be categorised as additives as well as simple carbohydrates.

Additives

Colours, flavours, preservatives and any other ingredients manufactured in a lab, are all additives. Anything that has been added to natural food is lumped into this section right here. And, if you never read anything else in this book, but ensure your family is additive free, you'll have to be doing some serious food abusing to be unhealthy. It is really, really hard to be unhealthy once you are additive free.

The food section of this book has two underlying themes:

- Eat a balanced diet, and
- Eat real food.

Eating real food means avoiding fake food.

Fake food is over processed junk that looks like a kids plastic toy version of food. Think about single pack cheese slices - they look like toy cheese, right? Well, leave them in a cupboard for a few years and they still look the same - you've seen those pictures of a 10-year-old Big Mac that still looks the same? Additives.

Lets look at why additives even exist.

A man decides one day that he wants to sell apple juice. He could grow apples, but then he'd be a farmer. Farmers need land and time, and there are so many risks involved with farming.

If you've ever made your own apple juice at home, you'll realise that it doesn't have that same golden colour that store bought apple juices have. Homemade apple juice is actually brown and cloudy. Getting rid of the cloudiness is easy; you just have to sieve all the tiny apple bits out with a very high-pressure sieve.

Once you've done this, you'll find out that you are left with a little over half the apple juice you had before, but at least it's not cloudy - it is still brown though.

It's takes about 5 kilos of apples to make 1 litre of unclouded apple juice. Even at a very steep discount, the man can only buy apples for $1 per kilo. How then, do the apple juice makers make it so cheap?

Well, they too have the same problems, but their solutions are a little different. Instead of juicing all the apples, they just get a big ol' tanker of water and mix in some "apple flavour" - a chemical that has been made in a laboratory. Apple flavour tastes just like apple juice, but it's so much cheaper to buy and there are no hassles with farmers and apple prices and pests and cloudiness.

So your juice manufacturer has now got a tanker of water, flavoured like apple juice. But it's still clear, so he goes back to the chemical engineers and asks them for some colours. Just like the flavour, he just mixes in the right amount of each colour to make it golden, and boom - he's got water that tastes like apple juice and now looks like apple juice.

But he knows that even though it is flavoured like apple juice and looks like apple juice, his buyers won't drink it, because it still tastes like fake apple juice, so he consults his chemical engineers again and they suggest he just add sugar, because the body reacts well to sugar.

"But I want it to say *no added sugar*, and they laugh and tell him about high fructose corn syrup. It's sugar, but it doesn't have to be listed as sugar. In fact, it's fructose - so it's the same thing you get out of real apples - except its concentrated and highly addictive - so you can just control how much you want in your drink.

The food man goes back to his tanker and pours in the high fructose corn syrup. He tests his concoction and thinks that it tastes fantastic. In the time it takes him to think this, the high fructose corn syrup has entered his blood stream and he thinks - "I want some more. But first I'll make it sweeter."

So he adds more HFCS and it tastes so much sweeter. He's finally ready to sell it and approaches the supermarket buyers. They ask him what the shelf life is, and he really doesn't know - so he contacts his chemical engineers again, but before he does, he asks the buyer what it needs to be. "The longer the better, because it gives us a longer period of time to be able to sell it all."

The engineers tell him to come and get some preservatives - pour enough in there and they will kill any living thing that might want to oxidise with the HFCS. Don't worry, they say, the colours and flavours won't go off, they're chemicals, bacteria won't touch them.

What happens once his product is stocked on the shelf is another iteration into the non-food dimension. Supermarkets are extremely competitive, so his apple juice will be sitting right next to the rest of the apple juices, and he will now need to market the uniqueness of his product.

Here are his options:

- Change the flavour to make it stronger flavoured

- Change the colour to make it more appealing
- Add more HFCS to make it sweeter and more addictive
- Reduce the cost of the ingredients by buying cheaper versions of them - so he can be cheaper than the other apple   juice manufacturers.

He finds out that buyers are a little more health conscious nowadays, so he opts for the final solution - he makes his apple juice more apply by adding real apples. Not enough to make a difference to the flavour, or to affect the use by date - but just enough that he can put a big sticker on his box that says "made with real apples."

The general public doesn't need to know that it was only one apple per thousand litres. Technically, it is made with real apples.

Looking back through this example, can you see how additives are very useful in a competitive business? Here's another reason we didn't even mention, *consistency*. People want to know that if they buy apple juice from you, that it will taste the same every time. With traditionally squeezed apple juice, this is impossible. With chemical apple juice, it is easy to do - the ingredients don't change.

Do you also see any point that the apple juice man is thinking about your kids? He's added chemicals to his concoction to sell apple juice, to look after himself - not you and not your kids.

Additives are not made with you or your children's best interests at heart. They are made and used for one purpose – increased profit. Food is no longer food, it is a science.

From now on, when you look at the ingredients list on the back of a package, you should be asking yourself why each ingredient is in there; and who that ingredient is in there for. If it's not in there for you, then it won't be good for you. Download the app called *The Chemical Maze* for an extremely useful and eye opening shopping resource. Just type in the name or number of the additive and it will list all it's dangerous side effects for you.

The only person, who will make food with your children's best interest at heart, is you.

Milk

We always get a kick out of those mums who breastfeed their kids past about 2 years old. We've never had a child *want* to breastfeed past 6 months, so we can't really judge the mum because we're not in that situation.

Getting teeth is a good indication to us that the child is ready to start biting their food. Nipples aren't designed to be bitten or chewed. So what do *we* do? We give the kids cows milk.

Isn't it a little weirder that we would breastfeed from a completely different species? We're the only species on the planet that does it. But cow's milk is a fantastic source of protein. It has over 3 times the protein human milk has. So we guzzled it down until someone told us that it was bad.

When we heard that cows milk was bad, we changed to goat's milk, the gentler alternative. Because breastfeeding from an animal with a beard is so much better, right?

So what's the deal with dairy anyway, why all the fuss?

Lactose Intolerance

Well, we all know about lactose intolerance. Someone doesn't have enough of the enzyme that breaks down lactose (the sugar in milk); they just can't seem to digest it. Lactose intolerance has been accepted for years.

But lactose intolerance is not an exact science, because people have varying levels of intolerance. Recent research has proven that 1 in every 3 people is lactose intolerant. If you are Black, Mexican, Aboriginal, Islander, Jewish or Indian. 3 out of every 4 of you are intolerant. If you are of Asian descent, you're a one in 10 chance of being able to digest milk.

If you're white and you're excited, don't be. Because after childhood, 75% of people who were not lactose intolerant will be. You see, drinking milk makes your body slowly lose the capacity to digest it.

Calcium

The whole calcium debate has flawed research on both sides. Milk, for many years has been touted as the best way to get your Calcium, something that has been marketed and pushed by the dairy associations of course.

Recent research has linked milk consumption with the potential to reduce bone Calcium. These recent studies use broad statements like "The countries with the highest fracture rate on earth are the highest milk drinking countries." Which while true does not take into account other factors such as obesity rate, contact sports and structural variances in different populations. A 200kg NFL retiree is obviously going to have more force through his hips than a small Japanese businessman.

The second thing the anti-milk mob says is that milk is acidic. Calcium is a buffer, so when milk is consumed, the body will leech calcium out of the bones to make up for it's acidity. While all of this makes sense, most people consume a highly acidic diet overall; not just from milk. And, consider that Calcium is not the only buffer, and can be replaced easily.

Sunlight creates Vitamin D, which helps the absorption of Calcium. There is a fair bit of Vitamin D in milk too, but Vitamin D is like the key that opens the door. Without the key, you could be taking Calcium tablets for life and never actually absorb them. Interesting that fracture rates are higher for countries further away from the equator (less sun)?

We actually dismiss Calcium as a reason to have or to not have milk. But you may have a different opinion on it, and that's great!

By the way, Kale has very high levels of Vitamin D and Calcium too. So even if you do feel you need to increase Calcium in your kids, you don't have to get it from milk.

Pasteurising

Assuming you are not lactose intolerant, milk that comes directly out of the teat of a grass fed cow is actually really good for you. One of the major reasons is that milk contains a whole lot of good bacteria that can inhabit your intestine walls and keep you safe.

The law says that milk has to be pasteurised though.

It is illegal to sell milk for human consumption unless it has first been pasteurised. Interesting that there are no laws against selling energy drinks to children though…

Pasteurising milk is done on one of two ways - both involve heating it high enough to kill all of the goodness that you would be getting from your milk (probiotics are bacteria, good bacteria; but pasteurising kills them). Pasteurising milk also changes the chemical makeup of the milk in the same way that heating polyunsaturated fats changes them to something different.

Homogenising

Homogenising milk is what manufacturers do to make it all the same consistency - much like our apple juice manufacturer who has to make each bottle taste the same. Forcing it at very high pressure through a tiny hole homogenises milk. Homogenising breaks all the fat molecules down into much smaller pieces, but without the disease fighting goodness of naturally occurring short chain fatty acids.

Homogenised and pasteurised milk is closer to sugar than it is to milk - it is much easier to consume, but it is not that easy to digest properly. It also goes rancid much easier, but that is unless there is a preservative additive...

If we were to consume dairy, we would only have raw milk, which is illegal. So we opt for eating cheeses and yoghurts. We like the high protein content for growing kids, as well as the probiotics. Cheese is a lot easier for kids to eat than meat or Kale, so we will quite often include it in meals that need a bump in protein.

To find out if you, or your children have a dairy intolerance, just stay off dairy for a whole week. On day 7, drink a glass of milk. Within the next 30 minutes you'll know if your body has the capability to digest it properly or not. Trust me, you'll know.

Here are some things to look out for:

- Runny poo
- Lots of farting
- Swollen belly
- Tiredness

Soy

When we were kids, the trendy thing to do was to replace your milk with soymilk, since soy was a healthier alternative. Sounds good in theory...

Believe what you want about soy, because there is so much subterfuge and litigation behind this simple little bean that it is hard to decide on your version of the truth. The story goes like this:

In the U.S of A, there is a huge company called Monsanto. Monsanto makes Roundup, the stuff that kills weeds. One part of Monsanto's company is to genetically modify plants in a way as to make them trademarkeable. Soy is one such plant.

The scientists at Monsanto managed to create a genetically modified version of soy that was immune to the effects of Roundup. Imagine how exciting this would be for farmers, who could blanket spray for weeds, knowing that the crop they were growing was not going to be affected.

The anti Monsanto lobbyist want you to know that any soy product you now buy and consume is a derivative of Monsanto's original commercial gold mine, the Roundup resilient soy bean. The genetically modified soy bean. The Frankenstein bean.

Here's a list of all the bad things soy has been linked to:

- Firstly, Roundup is not washed off the bean – every bit of soy then has roundup on it. Roundup is waterproof.
- Soy oil is an Omega 6 oil, too much of it which can cause inflammation and other bad things.
- Hexane is used to extract soy oil. Hexane is used to make

glue, and has been proven to be long term toxic.

- Soybeans contain phytates, which block the absorption of minerals.

- Soy contains isoflavones that disrupt the endocrine system.

- The isoflavones in soy look to the body like oestrogen, so either block or activate oestrogen receptors.

- Disrupting the oestrogen receptors can cause mild disruptions of the menstrual cycle, enlarging of breast tissue (but not linked to breast cancer) and reduce sperm count in men.

- Not only does it disrupt oestrogen, but soy isoflavones disrupt the thyroid too; messing with metabolism

- Soy formula for kids has been proven to increase breast tissue in baby girls, as well as create early onset puberty.

- Soy formula causes a longer, more painful menstrual cycle when the girl has grown up.

- Soy contains high levels of Manganese, which causes neurological problems such as ADHD

- Soy also contains high levels of aluminium, which can really mess your kids up by affecting the cells and the DNA.

We've looked through all the research and the only positive research we found had been funded by the soy industry. Even without the Monsanto voodoo, and the terrible way in which they treat their farmers (watch a movie called *Food Matters* for more on Monsanto), we just think soy is too risky to include in a child's diet.

Gluten, wheat and other grains

There was a study done on the performance of professional athletes and glucose intake. We remember reading it and nothing new really stood out, except when the researchers listed the sample foods to be eaten.

When they said to test using straight glucose, these researchers suggested a slice of white bread, because white bread is turned into blood glucose almost immediately. Faster than table sugar, they said.

We did a little digging to see if it was in fact true, and it is. Table sugar is made of glucose and fructose, two different types of sugar molecule, both absorbed differently into the body. White bread only has glucose. Glucose doesn't need to change state once it's in the body, it is already glucose.

Anything that has been processed so much that it becomes a very fine white powder should be avoided. Wheat flour is very fine. So fine in fact that it makes you sneeze.

In his book, *Wheat Belly,* Dr William Davis says that the wheat we eat now has mutated so fast that our digestive systems haven't been able to keep up, and a good proportion of the western world has a wheat intolerance.

But forget the wheat related diseases linked to wheat, like celiac, rheumatoid arthritis, Hashimoto's, dermatitis and dementia for a minute. Wheat has a protein in it called gliadin. When digested, gliadin binds to morphine receptors, giving you that feeling of addictive happiness that only comes from eating wheat. So in the same way Soy isoflavones bind to oestrogen receptors, gliadin binds to morphine receptors.

Combine this wheat euphoria with the fact that wheat flour raises blood sugar almost instantly, and we can see why wheat is making people so fat! High blood sugar means high insulin. High insulin means voracious hunger. Wheat then messes with our appetite, because kids just want more of it. Adults want more if it too!

We always say to do your own research, and in the case of wheat, just like milk, we recommend eliminating it from your family's diet for some time to see if you notice a difference. The reason we recommend this is because wheat is a staple for Westerners. We've all been eating it since we came off the boob, so we don't even know if we are intolerant unless we stop eating it and observe the result.

Think about that for a minute. Breads, pastas, cereals, as well as most packaged products are chock made with wheat. When we introduce any new foods, we cautiously try a little bit to see if we have an intolerance, not with wheat.

How can you know if it is bad for you, if you've always had it? When you have a mozzie bite, the area around it swells up to protect you from the bite. This is called inflammation. A rolled ankle is the same thing, the area around the ankle swells up to immobilise it and protect it.

If you or your child has an intolerance to wheat, the entire gut system will be inflamed. You won't know this until you've stopped wheat for at least a week. Many people who quit wheat will lose up to 5kg of inflammation in the first couple of weeks.

Inflammation looks the same as fat; love handles, muffin tops and a pregnant looking gut! If your kids look like they have a fair bit of puppy fat, or a bit of a gut with thin arms, they may be inflamed from a wheat intolerance.

Once the inflammation drops, you'll notice an increase in energy. You know when you have a cold, you feel like you just need to 'sleep it off'? Well, for some of us, the body treats wheat just like the bugs that cause the cold, and we have this feeling every time we eat wheat, that we just want to 'sleep it off'.

Finally, you'll notice a marked improvement in your children's behaviour. Dr Davis says that eating wheat for many of us is like eating crushed glass. You know how mad you can get if you have an itch on your back you can't get to? Eating wheat makes your insides itchy, something you can't get to. Imagine what this is doing to your child's mood?

Please do your own research; you may find that your children don't seem to be affected by wheat. Don't rely on popular opinion. Go and get the prick tests for your kids, because there are so many more foods they may be allergic or intolerant to. It is so handy to just know.

Be warned thought that the prick test only tests for gluten intolerance. It won't tell you if your child has a euphoric response to wheat, you will be able to assess this yourself.

Part 2:
Exercise

Is exercise really that important?

A few years ago, a lady came to us inspired by the Mooloolaba triathlon. Every year, she would watch the athletes run past her balcony, and at age 35, she decided she wanted to try it.

After talking to Georgie for a little while, we discovered that she had 7 older brothers. She was the only daughter of a farmer, and she was the youngest. Her mother decided that it was safest to keep her inside, playing with dolls.

Georgie never played with her brothers and never played outside. She grew up, went to university, got married and led a very 'lady-like' lifestyle. She never exercised and never went to the gym.

Georgie was not fat; in fact she had the tall, slim build of a catwalk model. Georgie's brothers all still play competitive sport. Exercising between 1 and 4 hours per day; every single day. 3 of Georgie's brothers are overweight, bordering obese.

You'll notice that this book is filled with nutritional advice, but we're only now touching on exercise. That's because exercise forms a much smaller role in making kids fat, compared to food. The old saying of "you can't out-train a shitty diet" holds true. Slim Georgie and her fat brothers are testament to this.

The story doesn't end there, because Georgie wanted to complete a triathlon. 1.5km swim, 40km bike ride and 10km run. After the first day, we realised Georgie was in trouble. Georgie had never learnt how to swim. Georgie had also never learnt how to ride a bike. But most troubling of all was that Georgie had never learnt how to run.

Imagine that! We all take running for granted, it's just something we have done as kids; many people have not run much since leaving school, but they at least know the feeling of it, they've experience it. Once you know how to run, you know how to run. Georgie didn't know how to run.

Teaching Georgie to run was like teaching someone a new language. Kids learn new languages really easily; but to learn a new language at the age of 35 is all but impossible. Learning to run, for Georgie, was like learning Russian.

Georgie is an anomaly, one person from her entire generation who never learnt the basic skills of running, climbing, swimming and bike riding. One in a million.

Josh, our eldest son, has just graduated from high school. In his age group, he can name over 30 friends who have never exercised. Kids who have never run or ridden a bike. 30 kids, out of about 100 that he knows directly. 30% of that small population cannot exercise.

Why has this happened?

It is hard to isolate a single blame point. Computers, TV, danger from playing outside, sport being voluntary at school, inactive parents. All these things add up to a sedentary life, a life devoid of exercise.

We all know that exercise is good for us on so many levels. But on a basic level, if you think about everything you actually enjoy - great music, making love, seeing a beautiful sunset, watching your children play… Everything you enjoy makes your heart race, makes you a little sweaty and makes you breathe faster. When you do things you love, you live on a higher level.

Exercise is like love. A daily dose of love, of pleasure, of unbridled joy. And it's free. Why would you not want to have a few moments of joy to yourself every single day?

30% of Josh's age group will never know the joy of exercise. 30% of Josh's class is destined for a life devoid of basic pleasure. They'll want it; everybody wants pleasure, wants happiness. So where are they going to get it from? A bottle? A needle?

Think about *that* for a minute…

What really scares us is that those 30% are going to have their own children one day. Who's going to teach their kids how to ride a bike? Who's going to teach them how to run? From birth, they will be surrounded by evidence that life should be lived slowly. Parents not used to exercise will tell them to calm down, slow down, sit down and be like me.

They may never actually say those words, but you've got kids, so you know how they just want to be like you. That scares us. Scares us so much, that we just had to write this book.

How to fix it

In our gym, we had so many mothers come through with their pre-school children. The kids would look forlorn and disgusted that mum had taken them away from the joys of the TV or computer screen. They'd sit on our couch, shoulders slumped, playing on mums smart phone.

Smart phones make dumb people. But that's a whole other story.

These kids would sit there each week; head slumped and completely immobile for the whole time mum was there. We told them they could go and play on our tennis court, or basketball court, or go and explore the grounds; but they would just mutter something incomprehensible and slump into the couch.

For about 3 weeks.

Then something amazing happened.

But before we tell you that, I better give you a bit of background. Most of these mums were overweight. Years of looking after kids and not themselves, they felt they just needed to finally do something for themselves. Besides, their kids were just zombies and they just didn't have the energy to change that.

They had tried taking them to playgrounds, bought them balls and skateboards and bicycles, but nothing had worked. It was so much easier to just park them in front of the TV; it's what the kids were asking for anyway!

But these mums cared too much to let it continue. That was when they called us, and we suggested *they* get fit.

Amazingly, on about week 3 of mum being there, the usually quiet child would lift their head and watch mum. At first for a little bit, then for much longer.

At about week 5, the child could no longer sit still. Long forgotten bikes, skateboards and balls all started to appear out of the boot of the car. Many times, the kids just wanted to join in with mum while she was getting fit.

You see, parents can try to push their kids into exercising, they can bribe them or threaten them; but this doesn't work against the lazy seduction of the computer game or TV. But if they get to see you exercising, and they witness the joy you radiate after exercising; they'll want in. You can spend years forcing your kids to do something they don't want to do, or you can take a few weeks to inspire them.

Kids are pre programmed to seek out adventure, fun and excitement. Your exercising is direct evidence that pure enjoyment is to be found and experienced outside of the rectangular screen.

Let us put it bluntly. You have a duty as a parent, to keep fit, and to do it in front of your kids. Only you; their hero, the love of their lives, can show them the joy of life. And there is no purer joy than exercise. Heart pounding, lung busting all out effort - nothing else on earth can block out the noise, can make everything make sense, can make you see yourself in pure truth.

Exercise. You have to do it for your kids.

What are the best exercises for kids?

Kids will want to do what you're doing. So if you're lifting weights, let them have a go - they'll be impressed that you can lift something they can't even budge. We certainly wouldn't start them on a weight-training program; it's way too boring for kids.

Plenty of people say that kids shouldn't lift weights, but we say that those people are looking at it with the wrong eyes. No kid is going to want to do something so boring, first of all. But more importantly, kids are much more athletic than we are, given their size.

Think about it. They climb jungle gyms and trees, they carry each other around, they crawl on hands and feet, and they run at full speed everywhere. Children are the real athletes. We shouldn't be trying to mould them into our boring way of training; we should be freeing ourselves with their way of exercise.

What does a kid call exercise?

Play.

If you're spending an hour a day at the gym, swap it for some quality playtime with your child. When last did you climb a tree? Play tag? Hide and seek is one helluva rush, but somewhere along the way, we all became too mature to play it. Instead we buy expensive contraptions to help us count to 10, for 3 sets, for each body part.

Kids don't count reps; they just go all out until they can no longer do it. They'll then sit down for a minute, catch their breath, and like a shot they'll be off again with a giggle and face splitting smile!

Kids don't need boring adult exercise; they need play. Adults need play too. It's free, it's exhilarating and it's better than any strength training exercise you've ever done.

On that note, kids love adventure and exploring. Instead of saying, "let's go for a walk" we say to the kids "who wants to go on an adventure?" Surely where you live there is a park, a botanic garden, a playground, a beach or a mountain. Take your kids there and exercise your bodies, as well as your imaginations.

Play is exercise, exercise is play. You're NEVER too old to play.

Sport

After about the age of 5, kids begin to yearn for more interaction. More fun, more excitement. Their capacity for physical exertion may have outgrown yours, which is a perfect time to introduce sport.

Don't let sport replace playtime with you; add it. Keeping up with your kids is a great way to stay fit. There is something mind blowingly empowering about playing a team sport with your grown up child. How old will you be when your child is 16? You need to be able to play sport with them then.

For you, for them, for your relationship.

Why your child should play sport

Sport is a phenomenal learning ground for being a better person. It's far closer to the reality of life than school is. Think about it, schools try to protect and handbag kids in an effort to breed a better culture, a more gentle culture.

Many schools opt for voluntary exercise, because kids might get hurt or picked on. Making sport and exercise optional is just as stupid as making Maths or English optional. It just doesn't make sense. "But obese kids will feel left out!" is the same as saying that kids with lower Math aptitude should sit it out. So they don't feel left out.

We would argue that Maths could be outsourced to a computer or a calculator. A person's health can't!

The pharmaceutical industry would beg to differ. "We'll look after your health... in a pill." It surprises us how many children are medicated these days. We know we're probably getting into some controversial ground here again, but when did we decide that our kids were to be brought up *dependent* on something else. A pill or a person?

Maybe we've been so heavily marketed to with the words *efficiency* and *outsource* that we believe the hype - giving someone else responsibility is true freedom, independence? What a load of crap. Taking full responsibility may be difficult, but it *is* freedom, it is *in*dependence.

When we were kids, everybody played sport. Without sounding all self righteously historical, we don't remember being hurt as something bad. If a kid rolled his ankle or broke his leg, he was celebrated for being tough; he took responsibility. Now days, kids grow up with no responsibility, so they blame. Often resorting to litigation. Since when is having a *victim* mindset useful?

Sport can be scary though, we totally agree. Sport is a stage where you set yourself up for being judged, set yourself up for losing, or for winning. But through your adult life, can you ever remember a time that you were not being judged by someone, where you were not competing?

Even if you work a comfortable job, you're still competing to keep it. Your employer is still judging you each review. Imagine if as a child, you got protected from the proving grounds of competition. Imagine if you never played sport.

There is a generation of kids in their early 20s right now who are testament to the damage that over protecting kids does. More damage than good. Our neighbour is 20 years old, a phenomenal boy. But he is the only boy we know of that age group who is not living with is parents, playing X-box and waiting for a career to fall into his lap.

Owning a gym, we got to meet many of Logan's friends. They'd come in with zero experience, and expect to be CEO. When asked employment questions, they would talk about themselves, not what they could offer. When asked pointed questions they would get teary. When given constructive criticism, they would storm out and 15 minutes later we'd get a phone call from their mother.

Not a realistic approach to adult life, you'd think?

Kids who are protected from sport and exercise are insulated from the real world. One day they will have to fend for themselves, we would rather they be well practiced in winning, losing, being coached and taking criticism.

We fear for the child who has been protected their whole life, fed dreams that "everybody is a winner," a child who enters the real world and finds it an unforgiving place where everybody wants to knock them down.

It's no wonder obesity abounds. Lets leave food and sport off the table for now. A child, who grows up under the protection of their mother and their school, will become so accustomed to being told *how* to be.

Once grown up, they will struggle with making their own decisions, and will so innocently crave the influence of someone else. In the outside world, the influencers are certainly not doing anything for the child's benefit.

Sport teaches kids to not only best their opponent, but to become aware of the tricks and games that the opponent will play on them. Learning to defend and attack. Learning to recognise subterfuge or trickery are skills of life, best learnt in the safety of a sports field, wouldn't you agree?

We could go on and on forever about the value of sport, but if you're reading this, you already get it. So we will move on.

When to introduce sport

While we love sport as a metaphor for life, there are some things to be aware of, for example trying to get young children to play organised sport. We tried ballet and soccer for our kids at a very young age.

It sounds like fun, the kids get their own uniforms and they look so cute. They get the chance to kick a ball or to dance around and to exercise, which is fantastic. But we have witnessed two very deep cracks in toddler sports that made us opt out completely.

Firstly, for too many parents put their kids into sport or dance so that they don't have to play with them. It is outsourcing something that you should be enjoying as a parent. But that's just our philosophy - we'd rather buy a soccer ball and play *with* our kids than to sit on the sideline like spectators.

Kids learn from us, they model themselves on us. If we're sitting on the sideline, they will think that is where they should be.

Secondly, we're not keen on the rigidity of toddler sport. Children are explorers, children love to express themselves - they want to explore their emotions and their body's capabilities. If they are constantly told what to do, or told to sit still while the coach explains something, they end up bored.

If you force a kid to sit still when they are bored, or if they are made to feel naughty for running away and exploring their surrounds, they will feel bad. Feeling bad when they are meant to have fun. That bad feeling can be subconsciously tied to sport for life.

And let's face it; toddler sport becomes more of a parent vs. parent event than anything. We were amazed at how many dads were wearing studded boots to toddler soccer. What??

It is our strong belief that unless your child shows a real passion for a sport or dancing at a very young age, you best to just play with them, or dance with them. It's a lot easier for you too, because scheduling toddler sport into your day can be quite disruptive, when they could just do it with you one-on-one attention; no standing in queues or sitting on their mats. Pure physical expression.

Stop when your child wants to stop. It may be only 3 minutes before they want to do something else, so do something else. Remember that they are explorers. It won't be long before they have their own schedules.

After about the age of 5, kids begin to yearn for more interaction. More fun, more excitement. You may not be able to keep up with their capacity any longer, or they may have outgrown your enthusiasm. This is the perfect time to introduce them to organised sport.

So let's discuss what type of sport is best for your child.

Team sports

What's the best sport for your child to play? Any sport that gives them joy; and no sport that makes them upset. Age 1-5, exercise and play should be about getting used to their bodies and the way that they can move.

By the age of 5, most kids have hopefully learnt how to ride a bike and a scooter. Kids should know how to swim, kids should be able to climb a tree, swing on a rope, kick and throw a ball. Finally, by the age of 5, your child should know how to run around, changing direction and speed; and most importantly; how to fall.

Many people forget that falling is actually a skill. A skill that is learnt only one way, by falling. Kids need to learn how to fall and how to get back up. Try not to prevent them from falling when they play and avoid making a big fuss when they do fall.

We have a friend who is always injuring himself when he rides his motorbike because he is a very awkward faller. He never really spent much time playing sport as a kid, so he never learnt how to fall safely. As a result, when he falls now, he looks like a thrown crab. Arms, ankles and collarbones smashed in crashes that should have just been rolled out of.

By 5, your child will be yearning for more interaction, and they have an inbuilt instinct to play/compete with people their own age. Every animal does it. If you watch documentaries, you'll see how lion cubs wrestle, chase and fight all day. They yearn for it, and so do your kids.

Team sports provide the perfect platform for learning about the real world. One team of kids join together to play against another team in friendly competition. Lets face it, unless you are in a gang, all your rivalries as an adult are with friends.

It is important then, to point out that sport is *played*. Sport is not war, it is a game. We'll get into show-mums and show-dads in a second, but please, please, please - don't burden your kids with your sport failures or family pride. Kids just want to have fun. They don't really care about winning, beyond the importance you put onto it.

When your children choose a sports team, find a sport or club that emphasises the joy of the game, not one that prides itself in its victories. We'd also steer clear of teams that overly emphasise the opposite extreme like "we don't keep score."

Find a balance, the best team for your child is one where the kids control the outcome. Be VERY careful of teams where the parents seem to be more emotionally involved than the kids. A good sign is a group of laughing, chatting parents, and a field of exhausted, but joyful faces ON BOTH SIDES.

Individual sports/ pursuits

While team sports emphasise community and teamwork, pursuits tend to teach kids a skill that is unique to individual sport... Responsibility.

We're not talking about "Johnny, I want you to be a responsible boy today" type of responsibility, rather a deep sense of self. Pursuits like swimming and athletics demonstrate to kids in a way no book, no teacher and no adult could ever teach them, that you, dear Johnny, are solely responsible for *your* outcome.

Not in a lonely, desolate kind of way, the type of responsibility you learn from sport is uplifting and empowering. Nothing teaches a child pride in the right things than working toward and achieving a goal.

Sport should be about fun

While we are able to talk candidly to you about the emotional benefits of sport and pursuits, it is more to make you aware of the benefits of sport, not something to coach into your kids. From a parent - child relationship perspective, it is important to be aware of the lessons being learnt so that you can help guide their thoughts the right way in an emotional outburst (and you will have outbursts!).

Your child doesn't need you to be their own personal Dalai Lama every time they come off the sports field; they just need you to be their friend.

Like we said before, kids work it out themselves - that is the beauty of sport - it is learning by experience. Kids learn to self-coach. It can be hard, but if you keep in the back of your mind that the purpose of parenting is to facilitate your child's independence, you'll realise that regaling them with your version of movie speeches just toots your own trumpet. Let them tell you where they went well, where they didn't. All you have to do is show them how much fun you have watching them.

Sport is about fun. And if anyone doubts you, get him or her to read sportsmen's autobiographies. Nearly every one will have a chapter about when they played their worst years. Nearly every one of them has a version of this sentence: "I had lost sight of why I played. It was only when I went back to the basics; to the fun of the sport, that I started to find success again."

Let your kids choose their sports

They could start with a sport *you* love, but we'd prefer you try something different by letting the kids choose. Go to a whole bunch of sign on days and let them pick. Don't feel pressured to sign up – sport clubs are volunteer organisations. There won't be crafty sales pitches, so it will be very easy to say no, or to just go away and think about it.

The reason we think you should try something different is so that you put yourself on the same level as your child. Let's say that you loved rugby. You know so much about rugby that you will want to spend hours with your child teaching them the game and making them better. They will never be as good as you or know as much as you, because you are older and stronger.

If you do choose to take your kid to a sport you played, just be aware if it, catch yourself if you find you are starting to get overly coachy or competitive. If your child is always being told how to improve or how to win, he could end up giving up. We don't want the child to play the game for us; we want them to play for the love of exercise.

Julius and his brothers are big rugby fans and all of them played competitively. When Josh decided he wanted to learn breakdancing, something Julius knows nothing about, their relationship flourished, because instead of a coach-student relationship, they had a team mate approach - when Josh learnt something new, he tried to teach it to Julius. When Julius messed it up, they both laughed - it was formative to Josh to witness Julius' comfortable attitude to failure; just like it was formative to Julius' parenting skills to be taught something by his own child.

Choosing a sport for your child that you know little about will make the whole experience an adventure for all of you. We really, really recommend you try it!

Quitting a sport

People put a lot of emphasis on quitting. "You don't quit on your team!" We disagree. Obviously, you don't want your kid to storm off the field through bad sportsmanship, but if there is a pattern of them just losing interest or not enjoying themselves, by all means, let them quit.

Life's too short to stick to something you don't enjoy, because you don't want to be known as a quitter. When Josh was 9 or so, he told us that he wanted to play on the same rugby team as his friends, which meant quitting the team he had been with for 3 years.

We asked him to explain the pros and cons and make a decision. He told us that team had lost sight of the joy of sport and was too focussed on winning. Parents had begun to yell at their kids from the sideline, even at practices. They were top of the table, and would win the season and he was going to quit for the bottom of the table team.

We had noticed that he, like the other boys had become seduced by the false love of winning. Aggression had replaced joy; the kids were stressed before the game; no longer cajoling one another and playing the fool.

I will point out that after puberty, stress from sport is a good thing, but only if kids have built a solid foundation that they can always return to. Sport gives joy. It is OK to be stressed, because you will always find the solution to any stressful situation is found in joy.

So we pulled Josh out and put him in the rival team with his friends. He immediately loved sport again. Joy was restored. As parents, we were worried about what would happen when he played against his old team. We should not have worried.

While some parents were yelling to "smash him" or to "kill him" all his friends from the old team still talked and laughed with him - even during the game.

Once again, evidence that the problem with kids' sport is parents.

Allow your kids to quit for the right reasons. Forget about your head trash around being "a quitter" and facilitate joy.

Find a balance

Sport for kids is about discovering a love of exercise, and learning about the outside world in a friendly, controlled environment. Children learn that excellence and self-expression is what makes sport more enjoyable, whilst learning that there are consequences to breaking rules.

Teamwork, sportsmanship, good losing, and good winning are all shared on the sports field, while responsibility; singular, individual, powerful responsibility can only be learnt through pursuits. Kids that have a pursuit become better team players, and team sports individualists learn the power of community and teamwork.

Just like food, it is important that your child grows up with a healthy balance of sports. Being seasonal forces this to be possible, but we suggest trying to find a pursuit and a team sport for each season. And to change it up at the child's request.

So for summer, you could do swimming as well as a skill based team sport such as dancing. In winter, you could have your child play some kind of field sport as well as an upper body power sport such as kayaking or rowing.

Can you see how such a split balances the child's body parts as well as skill vs. endurance vs. brawn? Summer sees an overall body workout (quite frankly, the best sport for children on many levels) in swimming, as well as a skill based, timing based thing sport as dancing (remember that dancing at this level is closer to a team sport than a pursuit).

In winter, there is a balance between a field sport - short, explosive running game with many directional changes, as well as an upper body endurance sport. Another great winter sport would be gymnastics, if you live in a place where kayaking would likely result in hypothermia.

Girl sport, boy sport

Until puberty, there is little difference between boys and girls athletically. After puberty, boys tend to get more aggressive and yearn for physical combat. This is the only reason boys should be segregated into a contact sport. It has to be their choice.

Don't make the mistake of putting your daughter into 'girls sports' and your son into 'boys sports' at a young age. Girls benefit from playing ball sports just as much as boys do. Learning how to kick, catch or throw a ball is a wonderful skill that once learnt, like riding a bike, is never forgotten.

Putting your boys into dancing lessons, just like music lessons, teaches them tempo and timing. Dancing and music are not just girl things. There are just as many male musicians and dancers as there are females. Wouldn't it be great if your child grew up knowing how to dance, so they didn't feel the need to get drunk one day to do it?

You will find among the greatest contact athletes on earth a high percentage of musically talented people. Team sports, like music, require a high level, subconscious awareness of timing and tempo.

Don't make the mistake of segregating your young children into sports or pursuits based on gender preference.

A parent's role in sport

Every parent dreams about his or her kid being the best sportsperson on the earth ever. And that's cool! Every time our kids play a sport, we see them in their national jersey, winning a trophy one day and dedicating it to us.

It's human nature to want the best for your child and it's a good thing that you are proud of them; they will feel that. But it is also very, very important to remember that their becoming an international sporting sensation has to come from within. No amount of pressure or coaching from you in these early years will make them champions. In fact, pushing kids at a young age has a high risk of damaging their future in the sport.

We've coached a lot of junior sport, and it always interests us to hear what each of the kids is doing when they grow up. Our experience is that the kids, who eventually quit the sport that they had so much talent in, were the ones with pushy parents.

Show parents, we call them. You know those people who dress their daughters up like dolls, and put them on stage to be judged against one another, beauty pageants for little girls? Imagine being judged about your personality and your looks at age 3 or 4!

What you notice from these pageants is that the children aren't competing, the mothers are. The mums. They have hissy fits out the back because their daughter wants to play with her friends and mum wants to touch up their makeup. Mum doesn't even see them as friends, she sees them as enemies, picking flaws in them, and reassuring her daughter that she is prettier with a tight smile.

These women are called show-mums. But they're not limited to the cheap hallways of American child beauty pageants. Oh no, the show-mum in this country doesn't live in a caravan and own a set of slutty wigs; she lives on the side of a sports field. And she in more likely to be a man than a woman.

The local show-dad storms the sideline of an under 6's match, wearing his own jersey pulled tightly over his swollen gut and screams at his child (or his child's team). He can be seen fist pumping when the team scores and he high fives all the other show-dads when his son scores. At half time, he can be seen stalking the orange bin, eyes feverish, waiting to pull his child aside and tell him what to do. Usually the advice is something selfish, like "don't pass it next time, just go yourself."

At the end of the game, Show-dad can be seen carrying his child on his shoulders (if the team won) or flat out ignoring his child until he can get him into the soundproof car, where he will yell and scream at him for playing so embarrassingly.

You see, show-mums and show-dads all have one thing in common, and it is the reason you never want to be known as one. Show-mums and show-dads never achieved anything in their sport, and are embarrassed by it.

These people falsely believe retribution will be found in the achievements of their children. So they push them and pressure them and drive them. All the while feeding their kid the same punch line "If I had the opportunities (parents) you had, I'd have been a superstar; you should be thankful."

Show-mums and show-dads live vicariously through their children. It is so much easier to drop the facade (because the only people who believe it are the other show-dads), and admit your shortcomings. Kids feed off honesty, and to tell them that you sucked at rugby because you were too scared of getting hurt, will make them better friends to you. God complex is not something you want to have around your children, and this is why we prefer to put our kids into sports we've got no emotional baggage with.

At this point, we would argue that everybody has a show-mum or show-dad inside. Where we all differ is how much of them we let the world see. The key point is to remember the purpose of junior sport; children need to experience the joy of exercise. Sport is the cure for junk food addiction.

Kids just want to be happy, right? Junk food always makes kids happy - it's been formulated that way. If they are being yelled at in sport, they will much more easily associate happiness with food, and failure with sport.

Flip the equation.

If kids find only joy from sport, they will have a split decision on their happiness. Sport makes them happy, and junk food makes them happy. It's an even fight. Hopefully in time they will see the ancillary results of each and choose their own path.

Being a show-mum or show-dad stacks the deck in favour of junk food.

Emphasise fun

So how do you combat your inner show-dad or mum?

First, be honest; tell your kids your own shortcomings. It's liberating and freeing for you, because most show-mums and dads had their own show-mums and dads. So tell your kids why you only ever played C grade.

At the same time, we recommend telling your parents why you never became the super star they wanted you to be. You'll be surprised at their response. Liberate yourself from your head trash.

Secondly, every time you feel the burn of show-parent coming up your throat, remind yourself that it's not about you. Sport is for kids to experience a joy of exercise. The real enemy is not the opposition; it is the junk food companies competing for your child's sense of happiness. They are doing everything they can to make customers for life.

Thirdly, emphasise the fun for your child. People *play* sport. Play is fun. Emphasise this for your kids. Parents tend to take sport way too seriously. Laugh before the game with your child, talk about how much fun it is to be playing the sport. During the game, keep your voice down because it's embarrassing. Laugh and cheer like part of the crowd, don't try to project your voice over the crowd.

At the end of the game, emphasise positive human qualities rather than winning, losing or innate skill. For example, instead of saying "you played so well," try "I noticed how hard you were working," or "you must have been practicing that move for ages," or "I love watching you because you have so much fun!"

We also think it's a great opportunity for kids to laugh at themselves. If they did do something funny, like miss a kick or drop a catch, laugh with them. Separate them from their mistake, and say "That was so funny how the ball just went the wrong way after you kicked it!" Or if they drop a ball, laugh and say, "You're so funny!" Mistakes should be embraced as a part of the game, not feared.

Predicting future success

Some parents will have read the last section and thought, "well that doesn't apply to me, my kid is special, he's going to make it. He plays representative level already."

Rep level sport at a young age can be misleading. Junior sport achievement is a very weak predictor of future success. Kids go through two sporting rebirths. Puberty levels the playing field in teenage years. The biggest, best kids get outgrown and the smallest kids can become gargantuan. After school finishes, priorities change and another huge reshuffling happens.

If your child does get selected for a rep team, try to avoid the "you are better than everyone else that's why you got in" attitude. Rep teams change from year to year based on position needs and unfortunately parent politics, so to make your kid feel like he is better than the rest can be quite hard to explain the next year, should he not get picked.

Picking your kid out to play for the country below the age of 18 is like gambling, you're playing a guessing game. We find it best to just focus, as we said, on the fun of the game. If your child is to become a mega star, it will be because he has done it himself, and because he has not been held back by anyone else.

Dealing with injury

Kids get hurt. It's a natural part of growing up, but there are two things you can do to mitigate the risk. Firstly, don't push them too hard. Ask your local physiotherapists or osteopaths how many childhood injuries could have been prevented had the parents allowed their child to rest.

Just like for adults, rest and recovery are where the growth actually happens. You can't train a kid to exhaustion, give them no time to regenerate, and expect them to improve. The problem though is that parents don't believe they are pushing their kids too hard until it is too late.

But there is a little test you can do to check if you are pushing your kid too hard. It's simple. For one week, do what they do. Exactly what they do. If they are doing 3 hours of swimming squad, followed by 2 hours of judo, do the same. At the end of the week, if you feel fresh, and revived, then you are not overtraining your child.

The second reason kids will get injured is if they advance through a program too fast. Gymnastics is a great example of this. We recommend going to a gymnastics teacher who is qualified to teach *progression*. If you go to a place that just teaches them the cool tricks, you risk injury. Progression is vital to mitigating future injury risk. Crawl before you can walk, walk before you can run.

Can you see how a focus on fun facilitates natural progression, while a focus on winning can tempt you or your child to skip a vital and risk injury?

Prevention is so much better than cure, but if your child unfortunately does get injured, a longer recovery period is better than a shorter one. It is very tempting to rush them back into their sport while still tender, but if you follow the doctor's guidelines and do the rehabilitation exercises, you will go a long way to preventing re-injury.

Re-injury is the enemy of confidence. Confidence allows professional athletes to take risks, the risks that make the difference between winning and losing. Re-injury introduces doubt and fear. Physical capability is not the greatest downfall of potential athletes, fear is. You will notice in your favourite sport that once an athlete gets injured more than once, their best days seem to be behind them.

It's best to think of your child as a lifetime athlete. A few extra weeks now can save them a lifetime of fear.

Lead from the front

Professional athletes are physical perfection. They are pinnacles of human physical potential. We all look up to them for inspiration. They show us what we are capable of.

If you were to ask a professional athlete how they got into their sport, nearly every single one of them will say that their parents were very active, and they just wanted to join them. Many professional sportsmen had parents who played sport, who took them to their own games, showed them how to be an athlete, how to behave. Showed them a joy for training, a joy for exercise.

These parents led from the front. If you want fit, healthy, happy kids; you should too.

Eat healthy food, and your kids will too. Train with an intensity that brings joy, and your kids will want to. Be happy, and your kids will too.

It's all up to you. You've been given a gift, you are solely responsible for the experiences of another human being, your son/ your daughter. You can give them a mediocre existence, or a powerful, self-affirming one. You are their conduit to a better life; you are their hero. Why? Because only *you* have the capacity and the responsibility to care for *your* child.

You are their world. One day, they will talk about their childhood. I hope for you that they talk about it with pride. They look back on the days with a tear in their eye and love in their heart. "I had the *best* childhood... my mum and dad were so inspiring, so instrumental in all my success... I love them so much..."

Part 3:
Reader Questions

Once we had finished writing the book you have just read, we asked our readers what their most pressing questions were. Most of the questions were directly answered in the chapters you have just read so there was no reason to include them in the book.

What we have included in this section were questions that just couldn't quite fit into the chapters and flow of the book, but were nonetheless important. We have also included some questions that we wanted to answer directly, rather than relying on what you may have learnt from the book.

Any questions that we did not answer by the time the book has gone to print, can be found here:

support.sharnyandjulius.com

Here goes.

My daughter does not like the look, smell or taste of red meat; is it OK for her to not be having red meat?

Of course it's OK, every person is different and as long as she is getting her macro balance from other food sources, red meat is unnecessary.

How much meat should children eat on a weekly basis?

Firstly, you need to ensure that your kids are having a balance of macronutrients (protein, fats and carbohydrates) in every meal. Meat only contains proteins and fats. An app such as *MyFitnessPal* would allow you look back through last week's meals to check that protein and fats were around 30% to 40% each.

If you find it higher or lower, you'll need to play with this week's food to either bring it up (add more meat while reducing starchy carb intake) or drop it down (reduce the meat intake). If you feel you need to drop it down, also consider increasing carbohydrates to match.

The second thing you need to take into account is your family's belief system around eating meat. If you choose not to eat meat, you will need to get protein from other sources. You will also find that there is a lot of protein in vegetables, so you generally won't have to supplement.

My 3 year old is always hungry. Should we let him keep eating forever (healthy stuff) or do we need to say no, kitchen's shut?

This is more of a parenting question, and it falls into the same category of "should my toddler be allowed to sleep in bed with me?" or "should I let my child eat in the car?" It's dangerous ground for us to offer an opinion, because it would just be that, an opinion.

As long as your child is eating healthy food, and I mean real healthy food, not food marketed as healthy, we don't see a physiological problem with allowing them to eat all day. In fact, preventing them from eating could make them have some future attachment issues to food.

In saying that, we have an open-fridge-open-pantry policy at home, where we allow our kids to get their own food if they feel like it. The problem for us is that it is hard to track their macros and it is a nightmare for keeping your house clean.

There are two important points to make here though. Firstly, we do have set meals; it's just that if they are hungry between meals, they are allowed to get their own food.

Secondly, and most importantly, having an open-fridge-open-pantry policy means that you cannot ever have anything in either place that you don't want your kids to eat. We use it as a way to keep ourselves accountable too, because it's not just the kids who sneak in there for a treat. You know who we're talking about, right?

How do I *know* if my child is eating a balanced diet?

In the book we covered how to introduce them to a balanced diet, using a macro-balancing app like *MyFitnessPal*, which is indispensable for checking their balance. Without tracking their macro intake, it is hard to find out if they are eating a balanced diet and whether that balance is right for them.

People tell us that once they have got their kids onto a balanced diet, they get told that their child "is so mature" a lot more often. As we said in the first part of the book, crazy behaviour is very often food related - either a macronutrient imbalance, or an additive intolerance.

What is the right portion size for a child?

Children are different to adults, because they are growing. Most children are hopefully far more active than their parents. Active children also benefit from a much higher metabolism, so as long as their plate is a balance of real foods like we discussed in the book, they may eat an entire dinner plate of food in a meal, or sometimes less than a cup of food the entire day.

Where portion size gets distorted is with processed foods. Processed foods, including all fine white powders, have a very high calorie density, as well as additives that mess with the feeling of being full.

A child's stomach is as big as their enclosed fist. A child's meal doesn't need to be any bigger than this. The stomach does stretch, and there will be times that your child will eat 3 to 4 times the size of his/her fist. Just be mindful if that is happening at every single meal.

Kids should only be eating more food than normal because of exercise, not because the food they eat is making them eat more.

Is it important for children to finish what's on their plates?

We don't recommend telling kids to finish their plate. It is not their responsibility to look after the starving kids in Africa by eating more food. It is your responsibility as the family CFO to ensure that wastage is reduced.

Many obese adults were told to finish their plates as children, and were made to feel like bad people for leaving any food on their plates. This feeling continued into adulthood when portion sizes increased and when they first started cooking for themselves. The mentality of "eating everything on your plate" is a big contributor to the current adult obesity epidemic.

"Saving the starving kids in Africa" can be thought of as a net gain equation. Allow your kids to leave the tiny bit of food on their plate now, so they don't overeat later. The amount they throw away now is minuscule compared to the amount they would overeat as adults.

Should children take supplements?

As a general rule, children should have no need to take supplements. If they are eating a balanced, unprocessed diet, they will struggle to be malnourished. The only reason a child should be taking supplements is if they have been diagnosed medically for a deficiency that they cannot correct with food.

And we mean *medically* diagnosed. Not diagnosed by uncle Vic or a friend from school. Doctors can do blood tests to determine whether your child has a deficiency. Uncle Vic or your friend from school may be right, but before you start putting foreign substances into your child's body, we recommend getting them professionally checked.

Once they have been diagnosed, by all means find a natural way to correct the deficiency,

For example, Himalayan sea salt actually contains almost all of the elements in the periodic table, so a pinch of it on dinner is equivalent to a multivitamin, but without the dangerous additives.

How does diet affect kids behaviour?

Behaviour (bad or good) is a product of the environment. A child exposed to parents who argue and yell at each other all day will be stressed and unbalanced. This stress and imbalance will display as bad behaviour either towards siblings or school friends or themselves.

If a child is exposed to a loving, caring environment where they are free to express themselves, they will mirror this in their favourable behaviour.

We could all agree then, that the environment children are exposed to affects their mood. What we forget though is that there is an *internal* environment as well.

The internal environment is not well protected. In fact it is designed to let everything in, unlike the external environment, which is designed to keep stuff out. The internal environment is far more sensitive. You could say that it was our Achilles heel, our weak spot.

Eating food that is bad for kids, even slightly bad for kids will display as bad behaviour. Slightly bad food can create headaches and stress, like watching mum and dad argue. Very bad food is unpredictable, like the behaviour of a physically abused child.

Food can be positive too. Nourishing the internal environment can have a profound effect on a child's behaviour in surprisingly wonderful ways. As we've said in the book, once you find your child's macro sweet spot, their behaviour takes on a more connected, powerful yet peaceful confidence.

Food doesn't only *affect* behaviour. For children, it *dictates* behaviour.

But, just like external behaviour, prolonged exposure can have a numbing effect. That is why adults don't bounce off the walls when they drink red cordial.

Is it a good thing to expose kids to junk food so they build a tolerance to it?

We don't think exposure is good, just like we don't think it a good thing to expose kids to crime so that they build a tolerance to it.

The final point on the food-behaviour link is that some kids have, just like external stimuli, a strong reaction to a particular internal stimuli or food (or in most cases a particular non-food). Just like some kids cringe at the sound of fingers on a chalkboard, some kids cringe internally when exposed to a certain food.

Most of the time it propagates as an allergic reaction, but without external symptoms, and to a lesser degree, some allergies are not picked up at all. It is only by vigilant examination of foods eaten that a parent can find out what foods their kids have an intolerance to.

Food intolerance doesn't have to only propagate physically. It can be diagnosed by changes in emotional state as well. And just like any allergy, it doesn't take much to set it off. Often a trace of a chemical is enough to start the emotional cascade.

How do I transition my kids from crap food to good food?

Basically this is a synopsis of the first part of the book. So here it is:

1. Create a weekly meal schedule, eliminating as many "what should we have" meals.
2. Shop online
3. Make sure your kids are hydrated
4. Prepare every meal with the aim to have each of the following: complex carbohydrates, simple carbohydrates, saturated fats, unsaturated fats and protein.
5. Remove all refined white powders
6. Remove all additives
7. Spend at least a month offering 3 -6 meals a day with balanced macros until they have corrected any imbalances (they will eat what they need)
8. Tweak the macros according to observation

That's the process; the reality is that people get stuck on the "removing all refined white powders" process. The best approach we find is to just rip it out like a Band-Aid. One day the kids wake up and there is absolutely no crap to be found in the house anywhere.

The fridge is stocked with fresh fruit and veggies and there is a wonderful, balanced meal on the table. School lunches are balanced and packed fuller than normal with healthy food and a few snacks from the book *Healthy Junk* and the rest of the day flows perfectly.

Why?

Because in the last few days, like an army general, you've planned your attack on the junk food. Every potential slip up has been mitigated and there is not a point in the day that your kids feel hungry.

That's the key - nobody should feel hungry at all. As soon as they feel hungry, the whole house of broccoli falls down.

Imagine you've only got one change to get this right. That's how you need to think of it. If you're not 100% ready, delay it another week. The little junk food junkie in them will look for weakness in you to leverage. The fight for junk food inside the little fella's head is fierce, and has to be met with a stone wall.

Don't get angry, don't argue, just offer more food (good food). Keep your resilience and eventually the tantrums will end, if you have any. Don't worry if the kids don't eat at all, they won't let themselves starve. Have plenty of good foods around, keep putting balanced meals on the table and they won't starve. A missed meal here and there is a small price to pay for your child's health.

Remember too, that you have to have integrity. You can't be hiding in the cupboard inhaling pieces of chocolate while your kids go cold turkey. You're a team who *must* beat this together.

The cookbooks we created called *Healthy Junk* are your saviour here. We created over 100 recipes for junk foods made healthy for you, without sacrificing taste. If your kid loves burgers, make him a *Healthy Junk* burger.

We swear to you it's worth it. And while you might think the tantrums will last forever, they rarely last more than a week. Be very careful of the sneaky ones. Older siblings, or spouses have resourceful ways to get their junk food fix. Get all older family members in on it first. Get their commitment, plan the attack and then commit. Go for it, you've only got one shot!

We have a 6yr old daughter who left to her own device would almost certainly try to survive on bread, biscuits and cake! The foods she will eat are so limited and I desperately want to open her eyes (and mouth!) to our great wide world of fresh, colourful and delicious fruit and vegetables. Her veggie intake is limited to pretty much carrots and peas so needless to say EVERY day there are carrots in her lunch box and most days they come home again…

Although she must eat them before she gets anything else! The only way I can get any fruit into her is baked into muffins urghhh! The only dinner that is NOT met with "yuck, I'm not eating that" is chicken nuggets or sausages! How do we encourage our little angel to nourish her body with the best fuel possible?

This is a great question, and we are pleased that you included the part about her gymnastics. If she were a sedentary child, I would recommend the above approach, but because she is so active, we can deduce a couple of things.

Firstly, if she is craving bread, biscuits and cake, then she is needing a lot of more energy from her food. Secondly, if she is eating only chicken nuggets or sausages for dinner, she is actually balancing her diet. High-energy carbs to fuel her active life, then high protein to repair and recover.

What we would recommend in this situation is, for a week; replace the sausages and chicken nuggets with higher fat content meat. Cheap mince is good for this. Giving her more fat, contrary to popular belief, would actually top up her slow burning energy stores.

What she's eating right now is actually equivalent to keeping a fire going by throwing in tissues. You need to throw in some big old slow burning logs for a while. Increase her fat content. If you want her to eat more veggies, fry some in coconut oil and top with a bit of salt. We can nearly guarantee that she will go crazy for the fat.

The cool thing about fat is that it signals the satiety buttons in the brain, kids eat for fuel first, then for wellness. Once she's used to being full, her body will begin to search out food that gives her a sense of wellness. Veggies and fruit. You'll probably recognise this yourself, if you've ever eaten too much fat, do you feel sick inside? What do you feel like?

Assuming you're not a soft drink addict, you'll almost always crave a bowl of veggies.

We'd give it a week to rebalance and a week to overcompensate (the fat) before you will see a difference in her eating. Once she's balanced her fat, replace the shitty carbs with sweet potato or pasta made from good ingredients, like quinoa. She'll still need the starchy carbs, if she's very active, you won't want to pull them back, but she won't need the highly processed junk; and she won't want it either, once she's recognised the improvement in her state.

The end goal for her is to have every meal balanced. She's currently bouncing between different macros, based on her last meal.

How do you go with birthday parties?

This was the most popular question by far, and a great question too, but the way.

For a long time we were never invited to birthday parties, I guess there is an ancillary benefit to being known as the fitness people. But we actually find birthday parties the absolute best setting for teaching your kids about junk food.

When we take our kids to a birthday party, we don't keep them away from the junk food, in fact we like it if they go crazy and eat as much of it as they can, and they will. Let us explain.

When Julius' mother was a child, she and a friend stole a couple of cigarettes from her father's study and smoked them behind the toilet block on her farm. Her mother caught the two girls and instead of rousing on them, gave them a whole packet and told them to smoke them all.

For the rest of the day, the two girls vomited and vomited. She and her friend never touched a cigarette ever again in their lives. The thought of it now, nearly 60 years on, still gives her a sore feeling in her stomach.

We obviously don't force feed our kids junk food, but if they were to overindulge at a party, and possibly vomit, we would take the opportunity to ask them about the food that they ate, and how it doesn't make them feel so good. Our kids go to parties now and either eat nothing, or seek out the healthy options. They are self-taught.

We also make a point of bringing something that they might like. You risk feeling like a bit of a dick if your child spews all over the jumping castle and the hosts hear you blaming their food!

A final note on parties, while Julius' grandmother prevented cigarette smoking for life, Julius' mother accidentally made her kids crave junk food. Julius' one brother Daniel makes a great example of this.

We'll let Julius explain.

Every time we would go to someone's party, mum would lecture us on what not to eat or drink and how to behave. Of course, when mum tells you what not to eat, you immediately want to find out why, especially if everyone else is eating it.

For Daniel, Grapetiser was the poison. Mum would remind him every time we went somewhere, "Daniel, stay away from the Grapetiser, it makes you sick."

Half an hour after arriving, he'd be complaining about a headache in the inside of his right eye (same place every time). Shortly after, a projectile, crimson vomit arced its way into the lawn.

Kids will always try to prove you wrong. Let them learn the lesson for themselves, let them make the decision as to what is wrong, and they will never forget it. They will own and defend that decision for life.

This doesn't just apply to birthday parties, one of our cousins can't stand the smell of cheap chocolate after an Easter binge when he was about 5, while Josh hates Haribo lollies (Actually we all do) owing to the way they turn your arse into a fire hydrant. For a good laugh, you should read the reviews for them on Amazon; you'll be rolling on the floor!

How do you handle food advertising?

If it were up to us, we would gun down every food marketing person in the street. Disgusting, slimy scum of the earth. We have a feeling that the food marketing slime jumped out of the cigarette sales barrel into the baby pool, where they resumed their evil work by seducing innocent children.

Junk food marketing is so much more than convincing someone to buy a product. It is about seducing them once, then hooking them with an addictive substance so that the junk food company have a customer (cash flow cow) for life.

How do *we* combat them?

We created our cookbook *Healthy Junk* to allow people an alternative to their addiction of choice. We also limit TV time. You'll be surprised how many TV advertising slots are dedicated to junk food. Modern technology makes it easy to download TV shows from the net, advert free.

The next thing we do is to call up our friends in politics, especially the ones with families and beg them to put a ban on junk food advertising, its like giving kids drugs and telling them that they are good; and this is happening on free to air TV (And bus stops, train stations, sidewalks) all the places that kids get to see them.

We also mention in this book, that you ensure kids have an alternative source of pleasure. This is why it is SO important to promote fun with sport, not pressure and competition. If the thought of sport brings stress to a child, then the happiness they seek (we all seek) is so easily found in a packet or a can.

Finally, we recommend buying all your groceries online and getting them delivered. The supermarket is rife with skulduggery and tricks to get your kids into junk. Why do you think the lolly packets with animals on them are on the bottom shelf? Because they're within reach of a child, and they know it's easier for you to buy the junk than it is to suffer a supermarket tantrum!

Buy online and make the marketers work harder for their upsell. You know their dirty tricks; let them try them on an adult, an even playing field. Every time we get order online, we have fun with it. "What cheap tricks are the marketers going to fire my way? If we buy into them, we lose; if we don't, they lose!"

How do you deal with grandparents and other family members that don't have the same views as you on healthy choices and feel they can give their grandkids "treats" and their response is "it is our right to spoil the child"?

Great question. We find that the reason grandparents do this is because they are of the generation that shows love with food. The first step is to communicate it to them, explain how Little Marcie behaves like a dragon when she eats junk food. If they still laugh you off like a little child, then remind them that while you are their child, they are just the in-laws to your spouse.

Good cop, bad cop. Tell them that if they keep pulling this shit, your spouse will prevent the kids ever coming out again.

If that doesn't work (probably because they hold some kind of financial or time power over you - i.e. you need them), we'd just teach them by experience, in much the same way as we teach the kids.

Organise for the kids to visit them, but ensure that Grandma and Grandpa look after them for the night. You *know* Grandma and Grandpa are going to do their damndest to make sure they are the favourites. Remember, they're cashed up with plenty of time; and believe us when we tell you; Granny vs. Granny is not sport; it's war.

The day of the visit, we'd make sure the kids spend all day watching TV and are really, really bored. "You can play outside when you get to Grandma's!" When you drop them off, make sure you do the right thing and leave them some *treats* "Its the least we could do," you say, biting back an evil laugh.

It's very important that the kids see what you've got them. Wise ol' Grandma is not to be underestimated. If that junk comes back with the kids, you're fucked. Get the kids enrolled - "If you be a good boy, grandma might give you some of these soon!" Leave quickly. Very quickly.

When you come back the next day, we guarantee the problem will be solved. One of them will smash some vases, another will probably tackle Grandpa, another will be like a dog who ate grass and drop piles of vomit on the Persian carpets. None of them will sleep.

"Those little guys have SO much energy!" is your cue for; "no, they're pretty well behaved normally, it must have been the food?"

In all seriousness, grandparents will come on board when you ask them sincerely enough. Explain to them how food is no longer food, and if they insist on treating the kids, please make sure it is made from natural ingredients and not chemical laden crap. Avoiding the obesity epidemic is a team effort.

Maybe get them to buy their own copy of *Healthy Junk* so they can spend some of their day cooking healthy treats for your little guys. Remember too, your parents come from the time where a balanced meal was actually the done thing, and other than the couple of small treats, I'm sure they'll be giving them a wonderfully balanced meal anyway.

How do you combat lunch box envy?

Firstly, we macro balance their lunch box with veggies, fruits, cold meats and some seeds or a half avocado for fat. But we've always done it this way, so realistically it would be hard to transition a child who is used to highly processed sugary crap to a green diet. Especially if other kids will tease them for having healthy parents.

That's why we created *Healthy Junk* so you can smooth the transition by substituting their usual junk food for the same things, only made from healthy, whole ingredients. While this is happening, we would introduce one healthy food option at a time. Sweaty broccoli is not a good option. Carrot sticks with guacamole is.

Slowly, you can swap out the *Healthy Junk* treats for more healthy options (hopefully you're well transitioned into a junk free home life). Within about 3 months, you child will not even remember his old lunch; unless you point out how much his food related behaviour has changed. Celebrate his successes with him.

Kids get it. It's very easy to try and trick them into healthy eating if you take the emphasis off taste. If you just point out the times where food-as-fuel or wellness is important, rather than asking, "is that yummy?" they will grow up with an understanding of food-mind-body connection that is inherent.

As far as dealing with kids being bullied for eating real food, deal with bullies the same way as you would for any positive trait bullying. Teach your kids to stick up for what they believe in. Be proud of their decision to be an individual and proud to care for their health.

When they are older, they will remember and talk to their friends about how they used to get picked on for eating *the same things every kid now has in his lunchbox*. They're front-runners, ahead of the game, and should be proud of themselves.

How do I hide vegetables?

Firstly, we don't believe in deceiving our kids. We don't want them to lie to us, so we like to live that example. Yes, it makes life difficult sometimes and there are plenty of occasions where it would be easier to just tell a little "white lie," but we are yet to come across a situation where honesty is best replaced with cunning subterfuge. But we don't work corporate jobs either!

The reason most kids don't eat veggies is because they have topped up their carbs with breads or pastas or some other starchy carb and they just don't need any more.

If you have a child who hates veggies, and you really want to hide them in their food because they just won't eat them otherwise, just remove all starchy carbs from their meals, and replace with veggies.

To ween them off refined white powder starch, make sweet potato mash and lightly mix the other veggies into it (as well as the meat). Sweet potato mash tastes so sweet, yet is so good for you, if you sprinkle some salt onto it, your kids will love it. Just be careful that they don't burn themselves, sweet potato holds heat much better than normal potato.

What starchy carbs do we avoid, and what do we replace them with?

Firstly, cut out any refined white powder (flours and sugars). Most of the dangerous starchy carbs are made with wheat flour, or have added sugar. So this means, all breads (including wholemeal and whole grain) all pastas and all cereals.

Replace these with lower calorie density foods that have higher nutritional value. Let's say your child eats Weetbix with milk every morning for breakfast. Try replacing it with oats (as long as they're not gluten intolerant) and a banana sliced into it. Use raw milk or coconut milk, then sprinkle some crushed seeds and yoghurt over the top.

Another example would be the spag bol for dinner. We would spiral zucchini and lightly boil it. Kids won't be able to tell the difference, but they will have the nutritional benefits of a green vegetable, with about a quarter of the calories, and no potential intolerance.

If your kids love white rice, quickly blend a cauliflower until it is rice-like and boil for much shorter than you would rice. Cauliflower is very low in absorbable calories, but high in nutrition. Once again, your kids won't notice the difference.

If your kids love sandwiches, make them a cheese and vegetable stack, just layer slices of cucumber, cheese and tomato to make a mini sandwich, without the bread. If they insist on having bread, you can make your own at home, we have a recipe for bread in *Healthy Junk*, as well as a banana bread recipe that is made with zucchini and banana flour, and tastes amazing.

When we finally realised that it was not cruel or strict to protect our kids from dangerous foods, we began to find creative ways to still keep the flavour, without the potential poisons.

Is gluten really that bad?

Gluten is only bad if your child has an intolerance to it. If you're concerned, you can get a prick test done at your local pharmacy. If the prick test is positive, you will need to eliminate all gluten-containing products from your child's diet.

This isn't such a bad thing. Gluten containing products are generally high in energy, but low in nutrition. Most people quit gluten, because it's easier than saying "I'm off bread, pasta, cereal and other wheat/gluten products because I can't control my eating with them, and they make me fat"

It's much easier to just say, "I'm gluten intolerant."

But to answer the question, if you don't have a gluten intolerance, then gluten is not the devil's food. There has been some recent research that links modern wheat to different ills such as ADHD and Alzheimer's, but that doesn't mean it is gluten. It's just that gluten is found in wheat, so if your family chooses not to eat wheat, it's just easier to say that you are gluten free.

As we've said in the book, be careful of blindly following diet trends. Do your own research.

Is sugar really that bad for you?

No, all carbohydrates are made of sugar. Fructose, the "bad" sugar is the sugar found in fruit. Fruit has been around for millions of years, obesity hasn't. Fruit is an important source of micronutrients for children and should not be eliminated from the diet.

Excess sugar is bad for you. If the only sugar your kids are getting is from fruit, then you have no problems. If they are eating anything processed, then they are more likely getting too much sugar.

Read the back of the packet to see if there has been any sugar added. Glucose, fructose, dextrose, high fructose corn syrup, HFCS, cornstarch maltodextrin, and anything 'syrup' are all words used to describe added sugar. To give you an example, all store bought bacon has added sugar. Weird, right?

Once again, be careful of diet trends. Do your own research.

What about PowerAde or Gatorade?

PowerAde and Gatorade used to be isotonic and good thirst quenchers. Profiteering got in the way and the companies that own them began to make them more sugary and with a ton of different artificial flavours.

Giving your kids PowerAde for sports is not advised. You can make your own version of it that will quench their thirst the way Gatorade originally intended.

In ½ a litre of water, mix half a teaspoon of Himalayan sea salt, juice of 3 lemons and tablespoon of dextrose (brewing sugar). Dextrose is just another name for glucose, and is absorbed straight away, and used as fuel without any changes in composition needed. Salt is an electrolyte and lost during physical exercise due to sweating (this is why your sweat tastes salty). Lemon juice adds flavour and cleans the palate; so your child doesn't feel like they're getting cottonmouth.

It tastes a little salty, but your kids will learn to love it, as their performance increases, and fatigue is delayed.

How do you stop kids from spending all day on their smart phones?

We don't see any reason why a child under the age of 12 should have a smart phone.

If you do have kids addicted to computer games or TV, just do what your parents did, restrict them to half an hour of TV at night, after they've been outside playing all afternoon. You're not a bad parent for facilitating physical exercise and imagination.

Julius calls it deadshitting. Sitting on a smart phone, with a dumb look on your face as you scroll through kilometres of social media. If you find your kids are always deadshitting, have a look to see where they are learning it from.

In our house, from 3pm to 7pm, we have non-negotiable family time. No phones, computers or TV. We are ALL forced to find tech free entertainment. Nothing calms crazy kids down more than being outside.

Do you think we need to have specific exercise time or program for young kids, or is outside active playtime enough?

Outside playtime should be enough. Structured exercise time is not a bad thing, but it's probably something you put into *your* schedule, rather than forcing the kids to play for exactly one hour outside. We would tend to just add up the active playtime during the day so see if they have enough.

To work out if your kids are getting enough physical active playtime, try to balance their emotional, physical and mental growth. What we mean is that they do need to spend time learning to strengthen their minds, which is just as important (not more important) than strengthening and learning about their bodies.

There is a third piece to the human puzzle, the emotional growth, which most people call the arts. Emotional growth is not just limited to art and music, though; emotional growth happens at the dinner table, when the family talks together.

Try to get equal amounts of each into your child's day to make them well rounded, mature adults.

Each of the three corners of development actually intersect. Playing music for example is great for emotional as well as mental growth. Playing make believe on a jungle gym is great for emotional, mental as well as physical growth.

Should kids lift weights?

Kids lift weight all the time, more than most adults. Think about how often a kid climbs up a tree or jungle gym. They are lifting their entire body weight. When they piggyback one another, they carry a friends' entire body weight on their back whilst running.

So if your kid shows an interest in lifting weights, let him try lifting a light weight – he probably just wants to copy your movements. If it's too heavy, he just won't lift it anyway – there is no way a kid will keep straining, and they should never be forced to. A broomstick is a great substitute for a barbell.

What about a structured exercise program?

We don't think it is necessary for kids in this age bracket. Structured exercise programs that focus on achievement rather than fun can be damaging to the child's perception of sport and exercise. It can become a chore.

It is our job as parents to facilitate fun exercise. By all means schedule your time slots to ensure *better* things don't get in the way, but if you feel you're becoming a little too militant about kids exercise, maybe try to be more fun. Crew cuts and burpees are not necessarily a long-term solution to kids health!

What would you do on a rainy day?

There are two ways to look at rainy days. Firstly, you can make a rainy day a rest day, which is not a bad idea at all. When rest-day becomes cheat-day becomes junk-food-free-for-all that this strategy turns against you.

The second way to look at rainy days is that rain is an added element to the fun. Rain doesn't make kids sick, staying wet for long periods of time does. So strap on some raincoats and gumboots and go for a puddle jumping exploration. If it's really raining hard, like it does where we live, get the boogie boards out and find some huge puddles for the kids to skid across.

Rain should not be a reason to stay inside. Our family LOVES rainy days because we will go outside and play in it, then come inside for a hot shower and clean clothes, before we dance around to music played really loud from the stereo. Dancing with kids is exhausting and so much fun!

At what age does correct technique become important for sports?

Technique is essential to sport and is the backbone of turning a sport into a passion. Golfers spend a lifetime improving technique. Tinkering with technique (assuming you know what good technique is) can be beneficial after around 6 years old; or when the child is able to understand that different technique will make them better able to enjoy their sport.

What you don't want is to be *correcting* technique, Correcting technique make the child feel like there is something inherently wrong with them that requires fixing. The way to approach technique is to ask the child if he'd like to learn a new trick that will make him faster/stronger/more efficient. Let them test it out for themselves and they will stick with it if it works for them.

Technique is something we find best left to professional coaches, especially with individual pursuits, where the lessons have been handed down and perfected for decades. Be careful that you're not being a show-dad or show-mum. If your child doesn't want to learn it, don't force it.

If you are worried that your child's technique may be dangerous, have a word to their coach - a lot of kid's sport relies on overworked, volunteer coaches who do it for the absolute love of the sport.

Kids surround them all day, and your child can sometimes blend in with the masses. Bringing attention to a potential safety issue is well worth it. Just don't hang around telling the coach how awesome your child is, or how awesome you were. You'll just become background noise again.

How much is too much sport or exercise?

We had numerous questions on this topic, ranging from parents of national level gymnasts to parents who are worried that walking their kids to school may be too much.

If you are asking this question, then we think you already know the answer.

You either feel like you are pushing them too hard, or as in the case of walking them to school, someone else is making himself or herself feel better by telling you that you're pushing them too hard.

If you feel in your gut that they're OK, then they probably are. Walking

2km to school is so much better for you and your child than riding in a car, listening to commercial radio.

If you feel in your gut that you may be pushing them too hard, give them a full week off.

Kids crave exercise and growth. Schools teach around 4 hours of brain work a day, so to balance it out, your kids *can* exercise and play for a good 4 hours a day as well. As long as they are eating well and the exercise isn't affecting the rest of their lives (falling asleep in school, loss of appetite, stunted growth), just monitor them for signs of fatigue.

Before kids are old enough for school, they spend almost all day running, playing and climbing. Adding it up amounts to around 8 hours a day. Just be warned that if you start them off on 6 hours of play a day, after a lifetime of sitting on the couch playing X-box, they will probably not move off the couch again.

The risk you do face with too much exercise is that kids will end up hating exercise. Competitive swimmers train sometimes 3 hours a day *and* play sport in school; many young swimmers grow to hate the pool.

To give a more succinct answer to your question, up until the age of 5, kids can spend all day playing. After age 5, until they start structured, high intensity sport, they should match their mental learning time with playtime. This is why we don't allow our kids to do homework until high school.

If like us, you believe homework is unnecessary, tell your child's teacher you will no longer be permitting it at home. Then tell your child that they will only have to do homework if they don't pay attention in school. An active child is a rounded, more intelligent child. A child that can silo their day.

Many times with Josh growing up, he'd spend the day at school and then come home to a mountain of homework that would drag on past dinnertime. This is not a balanced life. Kids need physical growth and emotional growth *as much as* they need mental growth. The body carries the mind. Sound body, sound mind.

Once your kids start structured, high intensity sport, they will need some recovery time. Recovery time is not Xbox time; it is time spent goofing off outside, playing in a playground, playing music, going for a walk or riding a bike. Anything where the children can manage their own intensity. If your child spends the entire time outside asleep under a tree, then you know they're exercising too much.

How do I discuss this with my overweight child without her feeling like she is fat?

This is a great question, and probably the main reason most people just don't make the leap into healthy living. It's much easier to just keep on going the way we have been going than it is to change, potentially scarring the child emotionally.

If your kid is overweight, you'll know this pain and this fear. It is the reason prevention is so much better than cure - this conversation is very touchy, and must be treated delicately. If you can avoid ever letting your kids get fat, you will never have to have this conversation.

But, if your child is overweight, don't worry. It's not nearly as bad as your think. There are a few things you need to know before tackling the issue.

If your child is overweight, they already know it

You probably put more importance on the issue than they have

They will only get stressed out if you overreact

- Body fat is inactive tissue; it's like a layer of clothing that can be taken off. Body fat is not something you can own, so saying "I am fat" is actually non-sensical. "I am carrying a layer of fat that I can take off" is much better. Separate *fat* from their identity. Saying it like this means that you can just drop the fat you're carrying, as opposed to becoming someone else.

- Overweight is a result of eating too much unhealthy food and spending too little time being active.

- Being thin is a result of eating enough healthy food and spending time being active.

- Focussing on the cause, rather than the symptom is much better, once again you want to separate body fat from identity.

- Getting them to lose the weight will need a team effort. You have to play with them outside and you have to eat with them. Kids become plump because they eat what you eat. Kids become healthy again because they eat what you eat; so eat the exact same meals as your child. Don't eat junk around them.

- If you make losing weight a chore or a goal, your child will hate it. If you make having fun the goal, your child will become healthy in no time.

- It often helps to show kids that *your* weight may have fluctuated throughout your life. Take out the photo album and show them the times you carried a bit too much weight and the times you didn't. For the thinner photos, tell them what you were doing (usually sport of some kind) and emphasise how much fun you had.

Never talk about losing weight with kids. Talk about gaining health. For kids under the age of 12, you can say it's like finding super powers. They get it. And they change so much faster than you or I can. An overweight kid, given fun exercise and nourishing food with plenty of water, will drop the puppy fat in a couple of weeks.

How do I deal with my child being called fat?

Kids get picked on for everything. Being too skinny, being too fat, being too white, being too black, being too fast, being too slow. Obviously you don't want your kid to be bullied, but let's face it; bullying is a fact of life. Uneducated, insecure people bully others. It goes without saying that we will never be able to eradicate bullying then.

So if your child comes home upset about being called fat; firstly understand that you will probably be more upset than they will be. So calm down. What you don't want is for the child to defend their fat.

So the best course of action would be to say, "Oh wow, I guess we have all been a little unhealthy lately, let's do something about it as a family so that you never have to be picked on again."

Remind the child that they are not their fat: "It is just like wearing an extra shirt under their skin; let's take it off because we've already got a school shirt on."

"How do you think we could go about fitting more exercise and better food into our week, son?" Be a team, he's not gotten fat; you've all gotten a little too comfortable. As a family, let's all have more fun! Stand together as a family, taking full responsibility against the bully, not against the fat.

Remember that you can make it a huge issue or a non-issue all depending on your reaction. If you nonchalantly reply with "Yeah, I suppose he's right. He's mean, but he's right; this family needs to have more FUN!" then the child will not put too much importance on it. If you go off your nut and ring the principal demanding retribution, you child will react similarly.

Carrying excess weight is not a good thing; and something that can be changed, unlike kids who get picked on for having red hair. If you're concerned about your child's weight and you've been wanting to find a sensitive way to bring it up to them, being called out at school is the answer you're after. You have a common enemy and you are working it out together.

You've got the child for life, and nobody really remembers the million things they got picked on for at school unless it was continuous. Get your family healthy, and they'll never be picked on for carrying weight again.

And on that note, some of the greatest athletes of our time, people with the best physiques, often comment about how they got picked on at school for being fat or being scrawny or being uncoordinated. Bullying can be a powerful motivator, as long as the child feels like he has his parents in his corner.

How do I handle my child being bullied for being fit and healthy?

We couldn't believe how many people said that their kid was being discriminated against at school for being too good at a sport, or too athletic, or too healthy. Not only by other kids, but by school teachers too.

One parent told us that their child got marked down in HPE (Health and Physical Education) because he didn't write a good enough essay on healthy eating, while the other kids did.

We'd like to stop it right there and say that in school, subjects are categorised as objective (the result your child gets is either right or wrong) or subjective (the mark your child gets is up to teacher discretion.) Now, no matter how objective a teacher is trying to be, if the subject is one that requires an essay, they cannot help but be swayed by their feelings for the child.

This is just like the real world, where someone's influence over another is directly proportional to how much the other person likes him or her. Everybody knows someone who defies logic by rising to a position they just don't deserve.

This is a great chance for parenting wisdom. Let's say your child gets a bad grade in HPE, and their essay is obviously not filled with grammatical errors and spelling mistakes, and you know that they are healthier than most of the class. Instead of calling the teacher an idiot and giving your child a superiority complex, talk to them about being more influential. Playing the game a bit, doing things to make the teacher like you more - this is far more important a skill to your future than formal essay writing. Being influential without being a suck up.

Obviously your child needs to know what they're talking about and we don't want a bunch of kids belittling the teacher; but subjective subjects are more like a delicate negotiation than the black and white objectiveness of mathematics or science.

What we're trying to say here is that your child should not be made to feel wrong, just like they should not be made to feel like the teacher is wrong. Where can you improve? Your essay may need to be a little more convincing or you probably could have done a bit more work off the ball.

Now getting back to your child being picked on for being too healthy. If you ask parents of overweight kids what they'd do if their kid was being bullied for being too fit or too healthy, they would tell you that they would dance around and probably high five their kids.

Which is what you should do. Because a bullying society breeds mediocrity. The worst thing you can aspire to be is just like everybody else. When your child comes home and tells you he is being bullied for being too smart or too athletic or anything else positive, cheer him on. Tell him that's awesome; go and find some older kids to play with, who are on the same level as you. It means he is excelling; it means he is breaking away from mediocrity and he needs to nurture that.

Many of the most successful adults we know match something they are good at, with passion for that thing. Just like many talented youngsters crushed their potential for the destructive ideal of "fitting in".

Tell your kids how the world works. During school, you're pressured to fit in (I mean, kids even wear school uniforms!) as soon as your child leaves school, it's a free for all and only people with something excellent about themselves actually excels. When kids leave school, fitting in is the last thing they want to do!

My daughter is just not into being active; she can't keep up with the other kids, so why bother?

This is every inspirational parent's dream. An underdog. Underdogs have heart! Tell your kids this; show them movies like Rocky, where the underdog wins through passion, hard work, consistency and determination.

Then ask her to what she needs to do to become a winner. Inspire, then empower. We're assuming she is school age, and that you are already on the journey to become a fit, healthy family; so underdog status is well worth nurturing.

If she is obese and just breaking stride is a huge effort for her, then a lot of work has to happen behind the scenes by you, her parents. As we've said right throughout the book; exercise should be fun, exercise should be play.

Even if you start by taking them to places that require them to walk around. Malls are great as long as you pack your own lunch, museums, zoos, and airports to see the planes, botanic gardens. Have fun, while you're there, maybe start up a game of cheeky tag, or climb a tree. What about throwing rocks into a lake?

Before you know it, she'll be fitter and stronger - just this little bit of improvement in health can be enough to make them realise that they can actually one day win. It just takes work. And work trumps talent every single time. Write that on the bathroom mirror!

How do I keep my kids immune system up during winter without resorting to the pharmaceutical crap advertised everywhere?

Day-care centres in winter seem to pass around bugs like crazy. Many parents say that their kids just spend the entire winter sick. Getting sick is a part of growing up, and a sign that the child's immune system is working.

Snotty noses are a sign that the body is getting rid of a bug. Snotty noses are not a problem, they're a symptom. Just like firemen aren't to blame for fires, they're just a sign that there is a fire and that it is being tended to.

But just like firemen, our immune system could always do with a bit of help, especially if the sickness seems to be getting out of control.

Our house is like a day-care and through winter it seems that just as one kid gets over his cold, the next is getting it. Obviously rest and plenty of water are most important. If your child just wants to lay down for the whole day, let him. It's part of him learning to listen to his own body.

We would encourage water drinking as much as possible, if your child drinks milk, water it down so that they are getting only 1/4 of the bottle milk, and the rest filled up with water. Offer them sips of water from their water bottle often. Offer them cups of decaf tea, or even mineral water. Water and rest cure most ills.

We have our own strategy for dealing with colds in our family. As soon as a child has the start of a cold, we give them a few ml of 5 mushroom extract as well as lots of water as described before. We use a steamer in their room with some eucalyptus and lavender oil in the water.

We also cut onions in half and lay them around their bed while they sleep. If nothing else, this has proven to be the most effective cold remedy. We also have a naturopath make up a concoction with eucalyptus in it and give the kids a dropper every hour or so if they are really sick.

We don't send them back to school until they have overcome the illness - it's like sending an injured child back into sport before they are fully healed. We've had a lot of illnesses over the years, but if we follow the above strategy, we've found the length of time and severity of illness to drop substantially. Touch wood!

To do your best to prevent illness, think about water. Stagnant water allows bugs to breed, fast flowing water does not. So most importantly, keep your kids weeing constantly. Because it's not hot, it is easy to dehydrate without knowing it.

What do you guys do when you eat out?

Eating out for a large family is expensive and quite stressful. When you factor in how long it takes to get served as well as food preferences, then add in 4 toddlers, it really is just easier to eat at home.

If you are going to eat out and you have the luxury of mature kids, then there are a lot of great restaurants that cater to healthy eating options. To stay safe, we would opt for the gluten free option or the paleo option.

Not because we think grains are the devils foods, but because we're wanting as much real food for our money as we can get. Breads and pastas are cheap fillers with very little nutritional value. If we're paying $30 for a meal, we want our money's worth of nutrition. When you focus on nutrition, volume and taste stop being your primary driver.

But in saying that, going out once in a while is a treat and if you have a healthy, junk free home, a good quality wood fired pizza can be enjoyed guilt free once in a while!

What are some easy ways to prevent emotional eating as an adult?

This is an interesting question and one close to our hearts. There are no scientific studies on the subject of emotional eating that we are aware of, but we have some theories.

- **Rewarding or bribing kids with food** connects food with doing well or being good. When kids get older, they may tend to be celebratory eaters. Celebratory eaters find it very hard to keep weight off when they lose it, because to celebrate, they want to eat!

  Kids aren't dogs, so reward them with something beneficial, like going to the zoo or going on an adventure. Just walking down the street is a nature adventure if you tell your kids it is!

- **Eating in the car** is an easy way to keep kids quiet, but it is very unhygienic and very hard to stop doing (we made this mistake). Eating in the car leads to this urge when older to stop in at a drive through and mindlessly eat, even if you are not hungry.

  If the kids are driving you crazy in the car, just pull over for a minute and calm them down. If you can't stop, just turn the music up loud enough to drown them out or play games with them to distract them like "spot the yellow car"

- **Eating around the house** sucks. If you can avoid it, please do. We made this mistake early on and like we said in the book, we've regretted it ever since. Every day feels like cleaning day. We do have an open fridge policy because we have no junk to hide, but we would have been much smarter to insist that kids only eat at the table. We're working on reversing this right now. Please wish us luck and speed!

- **Comforting kids with food** starts with boobie or bottle. It is very easy to calm a screaming child down with food. But unless they are hungry, this will only lead to comfort eating later in life.

- **Showing love with food** is another dangerous habit. Kids spell love T.I.M.E. The fastest way to a child's heart is not through their stomach, it is through giving them attention. Please don't fall into the trap of making them associate the feeling of being loved with tasty food. They are two completely different things.

What do I say to my child if she says she is fat?

It is vital that you disassociate fat from her identity. "*You* are not *fat*. Just like *you* are not *fingernails*. If you think you are carrying more fat than you want, then let's do something about it together."

Then just ask her what she wants to do about it. Don't make the mistake of saying, "Oh honey, you're not that fat" if she is unhealthy. She's come to you with the motivation to lose weight. Now empower her to make decisions about what they she wants to do.

If she is anorexic, you've got to speak to someone who can help. Anorexia is not the opposite of food addiction; it is a mental disorder that needs professional counselling.

Talk to us!

We'd love to hear from you, please let us know if and how this book has helped you. Just shoot us a quick email at

sharnyandjulius@sharnyandjulius.com

Thankyou for taking the time to read our book!

Sharny and Julius Kieser

You can also follow us on social media by searching:

sharnyandjulius

The Kiesers

Lightning Source UK Ltd.
Milton Keynes UK
UKHW020627311018
331512UK00013B/1300/P